ATTENTION DEFICIT DISORDER IN ADULTS

Third, Revised Edition

Dr. Lynn Weiss

Foreword by
Kenneth A. Bonnet, Ph.D.

TAYLOR PUBLISHING COMPANY
DALLAS, TEXAS

Also by Lynn Weiss

The Attention Deficit Disorder in Adults Workbook

ADD on the Job

Designed by Deborah Jackson-Jones

Published by   Taylor Publishing Company
                1550 West Mockingbird Lane
                Dallas, Texas 75235

Library of Congress Cataloging-in-Publication Data

Weiss, Lynn.
        Attention deficit disorder in adults / Lynn Weiss.
            p. cm.
        Includes bibliographical references.
        ISBN 0-87833-980-9 hardcover   — ISBN 0-87833-979-5 softcover
            1. Attention-deficit hyperactivity disorder—Popular works.
        2. Attention-deficit hyperactivity disorder — Age Factors.
        1. Title.
        RJ506.H9W445   1991
        616.85'95—dc20   91-28710
                                                            CIP

Printed in the United States of America

10   9   8

Acknowledgments

A big special thanks goes to my son, Mendel, who initially brought ADD to my attention as an eight-year-old child. He taught me to parent differently, and he motivated me to find out all that I could about ADD so he could have a good life.

Thanks to Aaron, my older son, who became an advocate for his brother and helped us understand what it's like to be a sibling of someone who has ADD attributes.

Dale Cheney, who helped with the writing of this project and who has become a good friend, deserves special acknowledgment. He learned more about ADD in adults than he may have ever dreamed existed and helped me arrange, condense, and write the many experiences that make up this book.

And thanks to Lora Cain, friend, colleague, and fan, who recognized that she had ADD from listening to me talk about it on the radio. Lora's generous input enriched this book immeasurably.

It is with appreciation that I acknowledge Mary Kelly, my editor, from whom I continue to learn each time we work. Her belief in the subject made this book possible.

A great big hug and sweet smile to all the people who have touched my life who have ADD as adults. This book is for you.

CONTENTS

▲

▼

Foreword

▼

The symptoms of Attention Deficit Disorder are compromising to the individual, and to the family and persons who work with that person. Attention Deficit Disorder is also a problem to the professionals asked to deal with it, and to the professional committees asked to establish diagnostic definitions and criteria. A large number of professionals are pressed by the individual client to diagnose and treat the problem, but there is little professional training to deal with the realities of the disorders and symptoms that are collectively referred to as Attention Deficit Disorder or ADD or ADHD (Attention Deficit Hyperactive Disorder). The narrow focus so often brought to bear on the individual with symptoms is that it only occurs in males, that they will outgrow it, and that Ritalin is the treatment of choice if treatment is to be undertaken. Methods of dealing with such symptoms currently include "time out," reprimanding, or stating that the individual with symptoms "needs to learn to . . ."; all are attempts to somehow coerce that person into "compliance."

The majority of symptoms subsumed under the concept of Attention Deficit Disorder are approached in the medical, psychological, educational, and family arenas with a very minimum of information about attention, attention focus, its anatomy, its mechanisms, its brain biochemical regulation, and its interaction with environmental conditions. This minimal

1

information is currently still reflected in nearly all aspects of the professional and parenting spheres, and more detailed information is often familiar only to the academician who has the least contact with the treatment or diagnosis of individuals with Attention Deficit Disorder.

Individuals with Attention Deficit Disorder may or may not also show hyperactive behaviors. They may or may not be male. Their disorder may or may not be evident to those around them. Some may simply miss bits and pieces of information presented to them that are assimilated in total by their peers in the same situation. The electrical, biochemical, anatomical, and developmental characteristics of the constellation of symptoms called Attention Deficit Disorder are now recognized as involving the central nervous system. An initiative developed by the Learning Disabilities Association of America resulted, two years later, in the report of the Interagency Committee on Learning Disabilities to the United States Congress in 1987. For the first time in federal language, the central nervous system is seen as having a major role in these symptoms.

The book you are about to read is for the nonprofessional individual. It is intended to provide the persons with ADD and those close to them with an understanding of the symptoms and their range and diversity. Dr. Lynn Weiss has accomplished this in an unusually effective manner. But she has also accomplished the accumulation of symptoms and means of dealing with them in a manner that can be very instructive to the professional who may otherwise rely on minimal information (unless he has personally lived with, or been very close to, an individual with Attention Deficit Disorder). Dr. Weiss provides personal vignettes that allow us to understand the daily manifestations and consequences of these symptoms. Reading these personal situations takes one far away from the simplistic views that an ADD person is a young boy running erratically around a classroom, symptomatic because he is "allergic" to one food chemical or another; that ADD is definitely/definitely not to be treated with Ritalin; and that ADD sufferers definitely "outgrow" their symptoms. These stereotypes

slip away as one reads the professional and personal information throughout this book.

The reader quickly comes to realize the full consequences of
problems with being able to maintain voluntarily focused attention on a task or situation in a systematic and sequential way.
These problems with attention may or may not be made worse
by certain chemicals or foodstuffs (individual sensitivities can
be severe), and they may or may not be accompanied by other
symptoms (including hyperactivity). For the professional, it
becomes very clear that ADD/ADHD is not a singular disorder,
and it does not fit existing diagnostic criteria in a large number
of cases. We must begin to take each of these symptoms seriously in the perspective of small but compromising deficits in attentional mechanisms rather than labeling them with an acronym
"ADD" that conjures up a reflexive and singular treatment
choice.

This book should be required reading for families, friends, and
individuals with Attention Deficit Disorder(s) who are inserted
into the human functioning of personal space and workplace. It
is also recommended as reading that may very well broaden the
understanding for the caring medical, psychological, or other
professional who has not had the experience of living with the
full ramifications of this cluster of symptoms. In the end, the
caring individual can improve his understanding of the person
with symptoms and through understanding can reduce the
stress he experiences in trying to interact with symptoms that
are not easily grasped nor fully understood.

Kenneth A. Bonnet, Ph.D.
Neuropsychologist, New York University
New York, New York
August 1991

Introduction

▼

I wish I had known twenty years ago what I know now. My expectations of my son and my husband would have been much different and more realistic.

When my son's fourth grade teacher told me, "He could do his work, if he'd just settle down," I began to realize that Attention Deficit Disorder was present in my family. Sadly, I didn't do much about it then. I didn't know what to do. Besides, I thought, as most psychotherapists and mental health professionals did then, that it would disappear when my son reached puberty.

It wasn't until my son was thirteen that my eyes were opened and I understood that ADD was a lifelong condition. My son's inability to block out the high level of activity in junior high caused him to become a frequent visitor to the principal's office. And he began to do poorly in math, the subject he had always done well at, because he couldn't concentrate on all the steps involved. I had him thoroughly evaluated for ADD and discovered he wasn't outgrowing it. In fact, far from disappearing, as we had expected it to, it was causing him more trouble, not less. And during the course of my son's evaluation, his father, by then my ex-husband, was evaluated as being ADD, too. It was then that I realized how ADD shapes personality, torments its victims, and fragments relationships. I did not yet realize the many positive ADD attributes. That came several years later.

At about the same time that I learned about my son and his father, two of my adult clinical psychotherapy patients failed to respond to treatment and I noticed attentional problems similar to those present in school children. When I went to the professional literature hoping to find alternative treatment for them, I discovered an article entitled, "The Diagnosis and Treatment of Attention Deficit Disorder, Residual Type," by David Woods, M.D., *Psychiatric Annals*, 16:1, January 1986, that outlined the condition in adults.

Then, on my radio talk show at KLIF in Dallas, Texas, I mentioned ADD in adults and its characteristics. I watched as the phone lines lit up instantly and the switchboard accumulated a record number of requests for further information. I soon found myself deluged with requests for information about ADD in adults.

But I had very little information to offer. In my research I'd discovered there was precious little available, and what was available was scientifically oriented and not helpful to the general public.

So I developed screening procedures, seminars, workshops, and group educational/counseling sessions. An announcement to the general public of any of these opportunities met with such enthusiastic response that all the available space was immediately filled. I was impressed with how eager those who have ADD as adults and their family members were to get help.

The emotional pain of adults with ADD became obvious immediately. But so too did their interest in doing something about their "condition." I began to hear the same stories over and over. And they sounded all too familiar. They were *my* family's story, too. Like termites that are unseen until the very structure of the building is jeopardized, ADD undermines the abilities and personality of the individual. Its damage spreads to the relationships that are an inevitable part of each person's life. And the pain is enormous. That's why there is such a need to raise awareness of this hidden disorder that, at least in part, can be held responsible for the way many people are. And that's why there's a need to develop materials and techniques to assist in circumventing the effects of ADD in adulthood.

My own son was placed on medication and given assistance in managing his ADD and at the end of the year won the citizenship award for most improved behavior. He passed algebra, too. With thoughtful, skillful help, he continued to be a happy, successful person who understood himself and his limitations and worked around them.

Nine years later this same son graduated from college. He's well adjusted socially and emotionally, and has learned to use his special kind of ADD wiring to his advantage. He knows who he is and feels good about himself. He's learned to cope with and seek accommodation for his ADD and knows what kinds of jobs and environments to place himself in to maximize his special ADD wiring.

One more addition needs to be made to this revision of *ADD in Adults*. When the book was first published in 1992, I thought that my son's father was the only source of his ADD. Only in 1993 did my own ADD become apparent to me. I am an example of a person who completely overcompensated for her ADD. Working all the time, I appeared to be a workaholic. But I wasn't. I was a person with ADD who had to work all the time to keep up.

I now know that many of the mental health problems of my early years were the result of obscuring my ADD. As I became mentally healthy, my ADD became more and more apparent. I also have come to realize that the special sensitivity and skills I possess are also a part of being ADD. And for that I am glad.

My intent for the readers of this book is to provide each with the same hope and opportunity for a happy, successful life despite the presence of ADD.

I have made no attempt to be inclusive. Rather, I am sharing what I have discovered works with the many hundreds of ADD adults whom I have treated and known. The names in the book have been changed, but the situations are real. I want to give you a sense of what Attention Deficit Disorder feels and looks like, what it's like to have it, and what it's like to be around it. And, perhaps most important, I want to offer some very practical suggestions for what you can do about it.

◂∣◀∣◀∣ 1 ∣▶∣▶∣▸

Life with ADD: Personal Stories

▼

Jeremy's Story
▼

I remember my desk when I was a child. It was usually piled high with papers, toys—whatever I was working on. Once or twice a year my mother would make me clean it up, and it would feel so wonderful. Somehow I could have a new, fresh start. The fresh start would last maybe a day or two. Then I would start piling my homework on top of my desk and I'd think, oh no, here we go again. The homework would stop as soon as the desk was cluttered again. I had no idea what to do with the clutter. It seemed the best place to put it was on top of my desk.

Today, my office at home looks like my desk when I was a kid. I feel like it should be labeled a danger zone. It's so cluttered that when my son comes in, he trips on things. My wife, who's the complete opposite of me, doesn't want to look at it. She's embarrassed for people to see it. The fact that I've lived in that kind of environment for *ten years* seems ridiculous.

I feel ashamed. I'm frustrated as hell. I feel like I'm not a grownup yet. On days I have to do paperwork, I make myself sit at my desk and try to get organized. My desk is piled high. I pick up a bill, make it out, and start to put a stamp on it. But the stamps are next to the paper clip box and I think it should go in the desk, so I put it in the desk. And I see more pencils than I need, so I throw two of them out. Then the phone rings, and while I'm on the phone I start throwing out junk mail, and there are magazines on the desk, so I take them to the book-case. In the bookcase there's an old magazine I don't need any-more so I throw that away. Then I realize that the waste basket is full so I empty it. When I go outside to empty the waste bas-ket, I see that there's something going on in the kitchen, so I do something in there. It's like I'm following a trail from one thing to another.

I can't get anything done because I can't concentrate on any one task. I can't seem to determine that, OK, this is the time to get the file cabinet straightened out. My motivation is always crisis. What gets done is what has to get done. The invoices I have to send out to get paid get sent out. The bills I have to pay so the insurance company and the light company don't shut off ser-vices get paid. I'm always late for appointments. Bills get paid at the last moment, usually, like reports in school were done at the last minute. I pushed the limits then, and I still push the limits. But if I had my druthers, I wouldn't push the limits. I'd rather not file two extensions every year on my income tax.

But I seem to have no choice. I have a real lack of attention for things I'm not interested in. I have poor task completion and no organization. I seek immediate gratification with no long-term goals. I've got no goal setting at all, really; I can't even set them. I just kind of fell into photography; I never sat down and said, OK, I want to be a photographer.

My file cabinet symbolizes my inadequacy for me. Ten years ago I was going to straighten it out. Now, ten years later, the file cab-inet still isn't straightened out. Knowing that I can't organize my file cabinet—telling myself that I'm going to do it and know-ing that I can't—drives me nuts. It makes me feel like I don't have any control over my life. It makes me feel ashamed and inadequate. It makes me feel frustrated and helpless. How big a deal is it to organize a file cabinet? We're not talking about brain surgery.

From society's point of view, I have the potential to accomplish so much more with my life, and I've come to see myself as lazy because I can't do certain tasks. Now I let my wife make the major decisions in my life—whether to buy a house, whether to have kids, how many to have. I just feel like I have no control over my life. Most of the time it doesn't bother me. But sometimes I get angry, really angry, and it comes out uncontrollably at my wife and my professional associates in sarcasm and shouting. I wish I knew what to do.

Jeremy Southland

Ann's Story
▼

        I grew up not feeling very good about myself. In school, it was hard for me to stay on the subject or to finish anything. When I didn't finish my school work, I'd get spankings at home. Teachers would be on my back. They said I was such a good child—they couldn't understand it. And I tried so hard. I just couldn't finish anything. I couldn't concentrate. I couldn't take notes even if I really tried. I was distracted very easily by practically everything. If someone sneezed, I'd look at him and my mind would go off in a million directions. I'd look out the window, wondering why he had sneezed.

And my coordination wasn't good. When I was in the third grade, I got up to get a vase of flowers. I fell and spilled the water. I remember one time in art class we had to draw something. I really tried, but the teacher used mine as an example and said, "Look how bad hers is. She just goofed off." They used to hit me on the hands with a paddle because my handwriting was bad because I wrote so fast, even though I tried to slow down and write well. I was always walking fast and doing everything fast—just making a mess. There were so many things I couldn't do. People would say, "If you'd just try," but I was worn out from trying. It made me irritable. I felt like a failure.

The situation has persisted into adulthood. I'm very disorganized. Take housekeeping, for example. After dinner, when I start the dishes, I'll wash a little, then run and wipe off the table, wipe the cabinet, talk on the phone, and never get anything completed. I have to really concentrate and tell myself "You are going to get the dishes done." Then they get done, but I still get the urge to stop and go wash off the dining room table. Just like someone is pulling me. My closet and drawers are still a mess, just like when I was a kid.

What's really hard is to stay with any kind of paperwork—bills, for example. It's my husband's job to do the bills. If it were mine,

12

we'd probably be in jail. He said he was going to do it because I made such a mess out of it. When I apply for a job, it's really hard for me to fill out the application. It's hard for my mind to stay focused. Only recently at age forty-five have I been able to sit down and write a letter. I usually write small postcards.

I'm the most impulsive person in the world. It gets me in trouble. If I see something I know I shouldn't buy, I'll buy it anyway. Or, I'll say something that I know the minute it comes out of my mouth I'm going to regret. I can't keep it from coming out. It's just got to come out. It's like a little monster. I'm bad about interrupting people. It seems like I have to get out what I'm going to say in a hurry.

I wish I could just slow down and relax. I have problems sitting still. I cannot just sit for two hours drinking coffee. During TV commercials, I'm usually up fixing popcorn, getting something to drink, talking on the telephone, or wiping off the coffee table. People say I make them nervous, but I don't even realize I'm doing anything. That hurts my feelings. I don't want to be different.

My dream has always been to be some kind of counselor, but I felt like I wasn't college material, so I got married and had two children. I have a real estate license now. I don't know how I passed the test. I must have guessed right. What I like about selling is that I'm always on the move and I love people. I'm tuned into them. But I'm too sensitive to have a sense of humor. I think I have a thin skin. I get my feelings hurt easily. When that happens, I cry and go into my shell.

My mood swings from high to low. I either feel very good or very down. I feel up if the house looks good. If I get everything done that I think I should, it makes me feel good about myself. I feel responsible for a lot of people. If my husband is in a bad mood, or if things aren't going right for my kids, my mother, or my sister, I feel bad. I don't know what's wrong with me.

Ann Ridgley

13

Jack's Story
▼

I feel like I'm constantly building a house of cards, a very unstable structure. Other people can glue their cards together, but I can't. It's so hard to come to a firm decision because I don't trust myself to tell what is right, what is acceptable. And when I do reach a decision, it's after hemming and hawing around.

There's never a moment's peace. I feel like I'm always juggling things. When I'm dealing with a customer in my business, for example, establishing a relationship. If that customer gets mad, even though I may know it has nothing to do with me, I'm crushed. I always try to avoid the action that makes him mad. Second guessing runs my whole life.

That's what I mean by a house of cards. Other people could just shrug off the anger. I can't. I blame myself, usually. Or I blame someone else. Blame's a big part of my life. Things go wrong a thousand times a day. If I don't blame other people, I have to blame myself. Because of it, I've never developed self-esteem. I'm always seeing what's wrong and always critical of myself.

And if I'm continually running through life, building these houses of cards and making sure they don't fall down, when somebody else knocks them down, I'm enraged. But I only express my anger at home, where it's safe because someone loves me there. I can explode over little things and they allow that because they understand me.

I can take just so much of the daily pressures of life; then I go numb, physically and emotionally. I don't know what it's like not to be mentally tired. Life wears me out. I need to get away from it, and alcohol is a way. Sometimes I just need to get drunk. Sometimes I withdraw and fall into a depression. Other people don't understand, and because they don't, they think it's ridiculous. What dummy in his right mind is going to go through life doing this to himself?

14

It hurts so bad. How many times can I hit myself with a hammer? Other people seem able to just slough off things they don't want to feel. I can't. Everything's important. Internally, I have no stability. I don't know who is right and who is wrong. Once I make a decision, I feel like my back is to a wall. When my decision gets altered, I can't accept it. That's why I grew up with my parents saying "I can't tell you anything. You're so stubborn, you won't give an inch. Everything has got to be your way. You're self-centered." I don't know what I'm going to do.

Jack Cooper

Lisa's Story

▼

In the fourth grade there was a girl named Karla. She was so sweet. She could be quiet and she could sit still, and all her teachers loved her. She never even had to try to get people to like her.

My dream was to be like Karla. But I never even made it into the classroom. I was always acting up, getting into a fight with someone, not paying attention, and doing things that would take me off the task. I just wanted to be heard. At home I was the one everyone pointed at and said, "You're weird." I'd want to be just like everyone else, but someone would point out something about me they thought was weird, and I'd get upset.

It's still that way. I'm still learning how to shut out things that distract me. It's hard for me to stay on task. When I started as a DJ, I worked at a local station. There was so much going on that there was always something to keep my attention. I could keep focused on the tasks. But when I got promoted, I had technical assistants to do most of the tasks. It was then that I ran into trouble. I had less to do that held my attention so I found myself drifting off during the songs, since they were all I had to concentrate on.

Next, I got my own talk show. It was great being on the air because there was lots to do that would hold my attention. But preparing for the show was something else. I'd get distracted at home going through all the latest local and national newspapers because I couldn't concentrate on one story at a time.

It was a long time before I started booking guests in advance. I was always waiting until the last minute. I put it off because there were decisions to make. What if I made the wrong one? I have a lot of expectations—perfectionism—and I wanted things to be a certain way. What if I chose the wrong one? A part of me said, "I just won't make any decisions at all." I'm great at making schedules, but it's hard for me to stay on one.

16

I'm one of those people who are all of a sudden switching topics in a conversation. It leads to some bizarre conversations. I really treasure friends who can keep up with me. Some people just look at me like I'm crazy.

I feel like I'll never be at the same level everybody else is on. I'm always behind, in the sense that they can get on a path and travel that path and get to the end. Me, I'll go to the right, then to the left, and then I'll get back on the path. Eventually I'll get to the end, but I never travel a straight line. I feel that if I could travel a straight path, I would be farther ahead than I am. And I beat myself up because of it.

My world was too painful, so I got into a lot of stuff that I shouldn't have—to tone down the pain. I'm better now, but emotionally I still have to work with the pain. If someone says, "You're so outrageous," it may be a compliment, but I perceive it as "You're so weird," just like when I was a kid. That hurts. I have to ask what they mean. Is it good or bad? I still get angry, but not as angry as I used to. I don't try to be Karla anymore.

Lisa Connell

◂ ◂ ◀ 2 ▶ ▸ ▸

The Hidden Disorder

▼

*F*orty-two-year-old Jason had come to see me for treatment of chronic depression. After a half dozen visits, I could see that my usual ways of doing therapy weren't working as expected. He was placed on antidepressant medication for persistent depression after a psychiatric consultation, but he remained the ineffectual Jason I'd come to know. Most people would have shown an improvement by then, or I at least would have identified the cause of the distress.

But Jason had me stumped. I was becoming increasingly tense around him, and not just out of wounded professional pride. Physically, there was nothing smooth about Jason. He was restless during our meetings. He continually jiggled his foot and shifted his weight in his chair. His eyes darted around the room. His mind jumped, with no continuity, from one topic to another.

Though he was bright, educated, and seemingly well-socialized, Jason's self-esteem was extremely low. He felt, and I agreed, that he had not lived up to his potential. He was unable to organize his life. He shifted from one uncompleted business to another, and, in fact, demonstrated an inability to stick with any project or subject for long. His wife reported that he lacked follow-through even at intimate times.

Jason complained that he kept getting distracted from his personal goals by whatever was happening in his immediate environment. He couldn't screen out the things that didn't matter. On the way to write checks for his bills, he would be drawn to the window by a tweeting bird, and then he would notice the overgrown grass in the backyard, which required a trip to the gas station to get gas for the lawnmower, which would lead to a conversation with the station owner about his wife's operation, which turned the short trip into an afternoon expedition, leaving him little time to pay the bills, as he originally (and with good intentions) had set out to do, or to mow the lawn.

The world was a booming, buzzing, confusing place to Jason, and his relief was to run, literally. He had become a marathon runner, practicing almost daily, running until he was exhausted. Then, in this burnt-out state, he'd stop his fidgeting and fall asleep in front of the TV or within moments of going to bed.

Exploring his family history, I learned that Jason's parents had bailed him out of scrape after scrape, all caused by his seemingly irresponsible, undisciplined behavior. But he paid a high price for their assistance. He was always viewed as "poor Jason" and "the black sheep." These were labels he couldn't escape. His wife had simply picked up where his parents had left off.

His mess of a life wasn't something that Jason felt he could do much about. No matter how hard he tried, he kept messing up. He had come to believe he was just a bad person.

He was wrong. As I watched him sit in his chair fidgeting, observed his short attention span and easy distractibility, and learned of his childhood disasters and compulsive need to run, I began to get a glimmer of what was going on. Finally, though it went against my professional training and everything I'd been taught, I tentatively diagnosed Jason as an adult suffering from untreated Attention Deficit Disorder.

▶ What is ADD?

Attention Deficit Disorder is a debilitating, little-recognized, and widespread condition that is surrounded by confusion and debate in the professional community. For decades, clinicians have believed that ADD disappears entirely with the onset of puberty. Others believed it declines in prevalence, disappearing in about half the cases. Now, a growing body of observation and research indicates that it is a lifelong condition, a belief which I hold strongly. I've watched my own son and other youths reach late adolescence with their ADD intact.

Like Jason, the adult with unrecognized ADD may typically be a mass of unfinished tasks, broken promises, and unfulfilled potential, subject to uncontrollable temper outbursts, fidgeting, resistance to being touched, and a tendency toward drug and alcohol abuse or other compulsive behavior. His behavior both creates and expresses a deep frustration and confusion, and a fearful sense of not being in control of his life.

The ADD adults with whom I work complain of an inability to cope with the stresses of life. They complain of chronic and unspecified emotional pain, and, like Jason, they may experience deep depression over their unfulfilled potential. Their frustration and uncontrolled temper may show up as child or spouse abuse or be expressed in other inappropriate ways. Friendships and family relationships are rocky and often fail.

Official definitions of ADD are developed by the American Psychiatric Association and published in the *Diagnostic and Statistical Manual*. As a result of new information based on research, clinical observation, and personal reports, the criteria for ADD is constantly being revised. In the appendix, page 158 is the current official DSM-IV criteria. The DSM will be modified from time to time as new information becomes available.

In the Appendices, you'll find a description of three types of ADD that I've found helpful for those of us trying to understand what it is and what to do about it. Following are characteristics common to most lists of ADD attributes:

► Difficulty with attention/focusing

► Difficulty with over-focusing

► Difficulty with activity level (hyperactivity, hypo-activity, or restlessness)

► Difficulty with impulsivity

► Difficulty with hyper-sensitivity (mood variability and reactiveness are affected by this attribute)

► Difficulty with organization of time, details and paperwork, or breaking projects into small segments

► Temper

From time to time, we all experience at least a mild form of each of these symptoms as we go through life. Occasionally we are distracted from the task at hand. In business meetings we may fidget a little as we long to get on with other projects that carry pressing deadlines. And none of us are strangers to bad moods, occasional impulsive gestures, or taking on a task without being well organized.

But, for the person who is ADD, it's not a matter of occasionally. It's a way of life—in a culture that demands all people to learn and perform in one way and one way only. As a result, ADD has been considered a disorder, when in reality it is only a different way of attending, focusing, organizing, and feeling. Most of the problematic ADD symptoms are secondary to being placed in an environment that doesn't fit.

Sometimes persons with ADD are able to constructively manage their behavior. They learn to work around it, and, in a few cases, to use it to their advantage, such as the high-powered, on-the-go salesperson or entrepreneur, or the comic who entertains nonstop.

More often, however, by adolescence many people with undiagnosed and untreated ADD have found drugs, alcohol, or other means to self-medicate or mask the symptoms of ADD, which often reappear after the removal of the masking substance or activity.

Even worse, many ADD adults, like Jason, are very strongly socialized to do "right," so much so that they begin to inhibit their behavior over all so that they won't draw criticism. They learn to hide their ADD. But, as with Jason, in the process they also hide much of their potential and become chronically depressed.

The attributes exhibited during childhood don't disappear. They simply take on a different guise.

Controlling temper—the result of high levels of sensitivity—is one of the areas in which adults with ADD often learn to mask problems. They may "control" their tempers in the setting that causes their anger, but display them later, at home for example. Consequently, seemingly small things can really set them off, and others wonder how they can be so irritable or angry. Yet their anger disappears as quickly as it appears; it is unlikely to persist day after day or week after week.

We know that all hyperactive children also are ADD (but not all children with ADD are hyperactive). While the hyperactivity may diminish, the motor restlessness that accompanies ADD may be more subdued, or it may be channeled differently. Like Jason, the adult with ADD may fidget almost constantly, tapping a finger, swinging a foot, or shifting his or her weight in a chair. Adults with ADD typically are a restless lot, always on the go, and they may not be able to relax unless they are dead tired. They're either going full-blast or they're nearly comatose. If they're not on the move, they may fall asleep almost immediately.

Adults with ADD most typically have poor attention when doing tasks not inherently interesting to them or when trying to do them in a way that doesn't fit them. But with activities they find interesting and fitting, their attention may be fine. This may sound like a failing in self-discipline, but it's not. Remember, they can be distracted easily by whatever is going on around them and are continually subjected to doing things they way non-ADD people do them. A non-ADD person would have the same type of problem if they were constantly pressed to do things that didn't fit them. Young adults, for example, are often able to write creatively and logically, but are not readily able to keep note cards and make outlines on paper.

Many ADD adults have difficulty sustaining a conversation with others, particularly in groups. Listening to verbal reports and lectures becomes overtaxing, and so they give up trying. Listening to stories that explain the process of what's being learned holds their attention. Because of the way most educational material is presented—in a non-ADD way—poor attention span can severely limit their intellectual and vocational achievements.

Poor impulse control in adults may express itself in their spending or drinking habits. They may be so-called impulse-buyers, often with dire financial consequences, and their impulsive approach to drinking can lead to chemical abuse. The "spur of the moment" is their constant goal. They may speak out of turn in conversation, seeming to interrupt without considering the feelings of others.

▶ How Many Americans Have ADD?

Professional estimates vary significantly, from 1% to 22% of the total population. That broad range never made sense to me. Now I understand why.

People fall on a continuum. At one end are those who do not have any ADD attributes. On the other end are those who have only ADD attributes. People in the middle of the continuum have half ADD and half non-ADD attributes. There is no one place on the continuum that suddenly makes a person ADD.

Whether a person is "diagnosed" with ADD depends largely on how well the person has found his fit in life, how well socialized he is, and whether he was trained from early on to develop his unique organizational, self-management, and attention skills. Learning to appropriately protect himself in relation to high levels of sensitivity will determine how well socialized he is.

Others' ADD-like characteristics are explained as drug and alcohol abuse, criminal behavior, or simply not trying hard enough. In all probability, the number of adults whose basic style of brain wiring is ADD may be far greater than generally suspected. I believe it is.

I have come to understand that ADD is a lifelong condition. You don't outgrow it. It never disappears. My own son reached adulthood with his ADD intact. His father, a practicing psychologist in his sixties, reached maturity with his ADD intact. So have hundreds of other adults with whom I've worked. I have never seen anyone who was ADD in childhood who hasn't continued to be ADD in adulthood. Some have learned to compensate well and found their fits in life, but their styles of taking information in, integrating it, and expressing it never changes.

Another factor in our inability to get a better estimate is the lack of a "data bank" on ADD. The criminal justice system harbors many adults who are labeled "criminals" who may be untreated people who are ADD.

ADD is not difficult to diagnose, though some professionals make it seem complicated. It is not a diagnosis of exclusion. ADD as a form of basic brain wiring coexists with all kinds of assets and liabilities, talents and maladies.

Individuals may possess varying amounts of ADD attributes. There is no set percentage of these attributes that makes you ADD. But if you are in settings where these attributes are creating problems, then you are likely to be diagnosed with ADD. In some settings the attributes that make you a success may be your ADD attributes. However, because you're successful, you might not be diagnosed as having ADD.

▶ What Causes ADD?

No one knows yet. Research thus far demonstrates that there is not one simple answer. Rather, genetic influences tend to be interrelated with environmental factors, such as heavy metal (especially lead) toxicity. In this book, though, I'm not talking about Acquired ADD.

The 1980s provided research data that suggest some genetically transmitted neurochemical characteristics in the brain. Though author Dr. Alan Zametkin hesitates to use the word "cause," a study by scientists at the National Institute of Mental Health indicates that a specific brain "abnormality" has been found in people with hyperactivity. Their brains seem to be less active, especially in areas controlling concentration and impulsive behavior. The results were seen as an advance but not the final word.

Clinical Psychiatry News (August 1987) reported that a computerized EEG distinguished between Attention Deficit Disorder and depression, "providing compelling evidence that psychological dysfunction alone cannot explain many patients' conditions and that biological evaluation is necessary. . . . Something is physiologically wrong." Though I understand that an ADD brain is physiologically *different* from a non-ADD brain, I do not consider something to be wrong.

I do not view ADD as an abnormality. Neither do I see ADD as causing or automatically coexisting with behavior problems, such as oppositional-defiant behavior, or emotional difficulties, such as depression. Rather I view these as offshoots or secondary problems resulting from an ADD person living in a non-ADD culture. An ADD person is measured against non-ADD standards and is found to be different. The ADD person is also continuously barraged by non-ADD expectations throughout life. These create the secondary problems that don't automatically have to be a part of an ADD person's life. The secondary problems don't need to be present.

In the 1980s and early 1990s, attention deficits were believed to represent signs of disorganized central nervous system function due to environment and social factors. Today, as judgments by non-ADD researchers are removed from the interpretations of their basic research, ADD can be seen for what it is—a neurobiochemical style of brain wiring that is neither better nor worse than a non-ADD style. It's not abnormal; it is only different.

For more information, consult the following sources, on which I have relied for this section:

Bonnet, Kenneth A., Ph.D. "Learning Disabilities: A Neurobiological Perspective in Humans," *Pro-Ed Journal*, 1989.

Coleman, William L., M.D., and Levine, Melvin D., M.D., "Attention Deficits in Adolescence: Description, Evaluation and Management." *Pediatrics in Review*, Vol. 9, No. 9, March 1988, p. 287.

Hussey, Hans R., M.D., "A Different Perspective on the Epidemiology of Psychiatric Disorder." Department of Psychiatry, University of Vermont College of Medicine, Burlington, Vermont.

Painter, Kim, "Brain Flaw Key to Hyper Children," *New Journal of Medicine*, November 15, 1990.

Clinical Psychiatry News, Vol. 15, No. 8, August, 1987.

▶ Who Has ADD?

Because the type of ADD talked about in this book is genetically transmitted, it is important that a family history be gathered for an accurate diagnosis: parents pass ADD on to their children. All classes and groups of people and all cultures exhibit ADD characteristics.

Originally, many more boys were thought to have ADD than girls. Now it is generally recognized that no sexual differences exist in the rates of ADD. Often, though, the behavioral characteristics are not as easily observed in women; are not as classic; or may be diagnosed as emotional, histrionic, or unstable behavior. Similarly, some less readily observable forms of ADD—particularly Form II, Inwardly Directed ADD (see appendix)—are harder for untrained clinicians to recognize and so go unnoticed.

▶ Why Be Concerned about ADD?

For each person directly affected by ADD, there are millions more—family and friends, employers and citizens—who experience difficulties, financially and emotionally, because of the lack of understanding of ADD attributes.

The high stress that unrecognized ADD creates often leads to addictions or excesses in all forms, including eating, spending, and working, that compromise the person's physical and mental health. After recovering from chemical abuse involving drugs or alcohol, abusers often demonstrate underlying ADD brain wiring. And the impulsive tendency of some people who lack appropriate guidance and education throughout their formative years are frequently mis-diagnosed as individuals with behavior problems without the realization of what underlies the problem behavior. It's like diagnosing someone with a fever and treating the fever without trying to discover what created the fever in the first place.

The educational process does not tend to fit ADD brain wiring. Therefore, children who are ADD often do not get a proper education and are considered poor students. Drop out rates tend to be higher for ADD youth than non-ADD adolescents.

In my practice I saw the ones who *are* bright. The others may have already dropped out of school and couldn't afford services. Studies of prison populations are beginning to indicate a high incidence of ADD—not because people who are ADD are more likely to be hardened criminals, but because of chemical abuse problems, untrained impulsive behavior, and low self-esteem.

For the employer, lost work days, increased insurance rates, and low morale are other consequences. Adults with ADD often change jobs frequently. One ADD adult I saw had twelve jobs in eight years. Some have more. This contributes to the high cost of unemployment insurance and to the high cost of doing business.

The family of an unrecognized ADD person suffers most, perhaps. Marital conflict, seemingly constant disruption in the household, and spouse or child abuse are all fall-out from trying to maintain relationships with an adult with unrecognized ADD. Codependency problems run rampant. The human heartache is enormous.

◄ ◄ ◄ 3 ► ► ►

The Abuse

▼

As a result of the "disorder's" obscurity, people with ADD are often scapegoats; misunderstood and mistreated. They go through life hearing comments like:

"She doesn't finish what she starts."

"He's irresponsible."

"She's smart, but just doesn't settle down."

"He never follows through."

"She won't let me comfort her when she's upset."

"He falls asleep watching TV the moment he comes home."

"She doesn't realize I'm tired, too."

"He's so immature."

The inference of this kind of comment is that the ADD person can "do it" if he just tries. Not so, or, at least, not without adjustment because of his ADD.

► What Causes This Abuse?

Words like *lazy, moody, unmotivated, irresponsible, too sensitive, clumsy, troublesome, insecure,* and *temperamental* are common in descriptions of adults with unrecognized ADD. Rarely are such characteristics recognized as only the result of neurochemistry that has never allowed the person satisfactory achievement or the luxury of living up to his potential. More commonly, the visible signs of ADD are seen as flaws in the behavior or even the moral fiber of the person.

▶ What Is Abuse?

To be abused means to be treated badly or unfairly, and, largely through misunderstanding, it happens to people with ADD physically, psychologically, and verbally.

Physical abuse (unless wretchedly out of control) is most easily understood by the victim and is the easiest to work with therapeutically. Psychological abuse puts the individual down and questions his self-worth and value, and is perniciously invasive. It convinces the person the abuse is deserved because of intrinsic wrongness within him. Psychological abuse is often experienced as the most confusing form of abuse because of its subtle nature; therefore, evidence of it is hardest to identify in the adult initially. Once identified, however, it can be dealt with, and early beliefs can be reprogrammed. Verbal abuse— name calling such as "dumb" or "clumsy"—gives the person a false identity. The individual soon comes to believe the labels to be accurate descriptions. Then they tend to live up to these labels. This is called the self-fulfilling prophecy. Psychotherapy can eradicate the sting of the hurtful words and replace them with supportive ones.

To understand how the abuse takes place and what forms it takes, let's start with the ADD person's experience from birth.

▶ Abuse of the Child

The abuse often begins when the person with ADD is a baby, and it comes in a subtle form: rejection. Because of their extreme sensitivity to touch and other external stimuli, the stroking, patting and jiggling that comforts many babies doesn't work very well with many ADD infants. Rocking the baby to sleep, usually a wonderful experience for parent and baby alike, may stimulate an ADD baby to waken. Parents can become just as edgy about being rejected as babies can, and so they may withdraw from their newborns when their overtures are rebuffed.

The abuse, again unintentional, may intensify as the child grows. It generally happens for several quite different reasons: The ADD individual finds himself in a culture that is designed along non-ADD lines. From his early years, he's taught and handled in ways that don't fit him—he fails and is then punished because he fails. The ADD child also does not receive training in a way that does fit him and from which he could grow and benefit. In addition, oversensitivity of the child means that he feels parents' and society's interventions more keenly than other children. Then, the child with ADD, laboring within an ill-fitting environment, reacts—creating more situations that bring adult attention and negative reinforcement.

Take Marcus, for example. At age nine, his life had been rapidly disintegrating, and not yet diagnosed as having ADD, he did not know why. He only knew that his inability to concentrate was bringing daily scoldings in the classroom, which were systematically eroding his self-esteem. He was also on the basketball team. Because of his sensitivity, he reacted to felt hurts. Seemingly impulsive, he was also losing esteem in the eyes of his teammates, and began to suffer from painful harassment that nine-year-olds are so good at handing out.

A well-socialized child, Marcus maintained control in the classroom, but by the time basketball practice rolled around, his control was just used up. One day, words mumbled under the breath of a fellow player, just loud enough for Marcus to hear, hit their mark. In a brief, uncontrolled moment, Marcus hurled his body at the boy who, unfortunately, tripped over his own growing feet, fell back, and bumped his head on a brick wall.

No doubt frightened by the obvious show of violence, the coach gave no thought to how it started, and Marcus got it—a loud, embarrassing scolding. And Marcus retaliated with rich words questioning the coach's ancestry.

Marcus was already frightened by the result of his own reactions. He had only meant to shove the kid to get him to shut up, not push his head into the wall. Then he felt further assaulted by the coach's words, trapped by misunderstanding—and alone. He did the only thing he knew how to do. He walked away. But even this he was later criticized for, because he did not "take his medicine."

Since Marcus could not control his behavior, the child felt quite victimized by the adult's negative attention. The incident left the marks of abuse—no one realized how badly this sensitive child hurt, day after day.

Parents, with the best intentions, just as unthinkingly may play their role in the abuse of their growing ADD child. Many parents want to be proud of their children, and equally natural to communicate that desire to them. We expect them to produce in school so we can feel acceptable, and we expect the ADD child to achieve by being taught in the same way as a non-ADD child in a classroom with twenty-five other children. But what about the child who cannot screen out external stimuli? What of the child who learns kinesthetically—through a hands-on approach rather than being told about the lesson? He's still told it's his responsibility to pay attention. When he doesn't, because he can't, the abuse may come in the form of well-meant scoldings or behavioral limits that the child can't abide—groundings or being kept after school. Of course, at times the abuse may be much more severe than that, from overreactive responses (remember, many children with ADD may have an undiagnosed parent who is also volatile, susceptible to frustration, and overreactive) such as groundings for weeks on end, to actual physical punishment.

Such abuse may rise from completely benign circumstances, but it's abuse nonetheless, and a legacy of scoldings and blame from teachers and parents remains for life. I don't mean to blame the teachers or parents. Their intent is good and decent, namely, to properly raise the child. But they become frustrated and don't know how to guide the child.

► The Legacy of Abuse

How does such childhood abuse show up in adults? Often, it takes the form of self-abuse, including low self-esteem, under achievement, and addictive behavior. Take Jennifer, who has been in an entry level, civil service position for five years despite having a college degree. She has low self-esteem and doesn't believe she's capable of doing any better. She was often told she was "dumb" and would only be able to do the simplest of jobs. This verbal abuse stunted her self-confidence. Or take George, a successful salesman who starts drinking every day at noon. As a child, he'd been labeled lazy and repeatedly punished at home and at school for not finishing his school work. Without alcohol, he felt the pain of the switchings and rapped knuckles and the anxiety of childhood every time he entered a place of business. George had been physically and emotionally abused.

► ADD and Procrastination

At times it seems that everyone—spouse, family, and employer—is angry with the adult with ADD, and all for the same reason: procrastination. It can be perceived as thoughtlessness or laziness, but it is still procrastination. The wife or husband feels that personal needs aren't being met. The employer doesn't understand why projects are incomplete, why deadlines are not met. The criticism isn't long in coming.

Procrastination, in reality, is many things, none of which is lazy or, necessarily, thoughtless. In therapy circles, procrastination is traditionally considered to be a learned fear response. It may be a response to trying to do what you should when you really don't want to do it (also called resistance). It may be rebellion against an authority figure. Sometimes it is a fear of failure, fear that work turned in will not be acceptable.

Such reasons are indeed sometimes valid explanations for ADD persons who put off work. Remember, they are more susceptible to the fear of failure than the general population, because they've often had more experience with failure. But, with the ADD profile in mind, consider another reason why they "appear" to procrastinate: Distractibility. They begin a project with good intentions and plenty of time, but they get distracted before they complete it. This only leads to more criticism from others, so that criticism and abuse haunt the person with undiagnosed ADD from infancy through childhood and on into adulthood.

Finally, what is called procrastination may be a misinterpretation of the way in which the ADD person works. But after being told year after year that they "procrastinate"—and that procrastinating is bad—they don't learn to accept their natural way of performing an assignment, which is different from their non-ADD counterparts.

◄ ┃◄┃ ◄ ┃ 4 ┃► ┃► ┃►

The Inner Pain

▼

*P*ersons with ADD often are excruciatingly aware of their inadequacies (though they can't identify their source).

They know perhaps better than anyone the discrepancy between their potential and the actual level of their performance. This knowledge is a source of intense pain. Like people in the cases we've seen so far, they understood what was expected in a classroom but not the way to do it that fit them. Usually, though, they were blamed for being wrong. Talk about helpless, gut-wrenching pain.

Later in life, as an adult, a person with ADD may have an idea that will solve his company's cash shortfall, but somehow he keeps getting distracted from mobilizing the information into the style of report his boss finds acceptable. Talk about frustration. You can feel it in the pit of your stomach. And it's doubly painful because he remembers the feeling from his childhood.

► Grief

The inability to live up to potential creates a sense of loss. And, like all losses in our lives, the loss of ability means we're in for the emotions of grief.

With grief, we normally go through several stages of emotion—denial, anger, bargaining, depression—that end with a healthy resolution: acceptance of our loss. After that, we go on to live full and happy lives. Often we need—and receive—assistance in working through our grief.

But in undiagnosed and untreated ADD persons, the grief has seldom been worked with because the loss hasn't been recognized. As a consequence, they may get caught up in the anger or depression that are a natural part of the loss and grief cycle. Originally, for people with ADD, the unresolved anger and depression may be felt only in relation to school work. Then they are likely to generalize to any learning situation or expected task. Finally, they may generalize even further, until they are angry or depressed all the time.

▶ Anger

Very often the emotion we see in persons with ADD is anger: Explosive tempers set off by seemingly small incidents—or no incident at all, at least in the eyes of others.

Persons with ADD suffer from anger for a variety of reasons, certainly, and unresolved grief is one of them. Another reason is that ADD makes a person less effective than he or she otherwise would be, which leads to frustration. And because ADD is beyond the control of the individual, there is a sense that life is out of control, which causes feelings of helplessness. Perhaps most important is the unrecognized sensitivity that leaves ADD people continually unprotected. Both frustration and helplessness hurt—a lot. And anger comes automatically as a defense against the hurt. But there's always some other feeling under the anger—helplessness, hopelessness, fear, or frustration.

▶ Flooding

There's another factor behind the anger we see in unresolved ADD—the emotional flooding persons with ADD experience.

The phrase "thin-skinned" was tailor-made for the ADD person. His emotional skin is paper-thin and does not block stimuli that come at him, nor does it deflect incoming particles of experience. Instead, his porous system absorbs instantly all that is in the environment, and the absorption is so fast and intense and pervasive that it "floods" the person.

The sensation of flooding threatens and confuses the person with ADD and he reacts—almost in desperation, as if to save his life, for that is how it feels to him.

He is aware of everything that's going on around him and "wears his feelings on his sleeve." Though often labeled overreactive, the ADD person really isn't, when we factor in his thin skin. He overreacts only by common standards, but considering the intensity of the feelings he experiences, his reactions make sense.

This vulnerability to hurt leaves the person with ADD in need of protection which often takes the form of temper outbursts and striking out over the slightest thing. "Push away the hurt" says the outburst. Often, the cause of the outburst is overlooked, but it's always there. A defense? You bet, and much needed until the person can develop other, more effective defenses with fewer side effects.

▶ Confusion

In a person with untreated ADD, you are likely to find the sadness of being blamed for not paying attention, the hurt of being scolded, put down, or even physically punished for work not done—because the work could not be done in the way expected. You may find the helplessness of not understanding what went wrong or what could have been done to change it. You may find, too, an utter hopelessness.

Often, however, you find confusion. "Why is she angry with me?" asks the husband. "I was doing the best I could." As in the case of the man who sets out to pay the bills and take his wife to dinner, but who ends up in conversation at the gas station while she's wondering where he is, the feeling is confusion. Why are you angry with me? Why can't I just concentrate on what I'm supposed to think about? Why can't I go from point A to point B without a lot of distractions? Why is my life such a mess?

Remember, people with undiagnosed and untreated ADD find the world a booming, buzzing place. They are unable to discipline their environment—to screen out the unwanted stimuli that invade their lives. And it's not just the world that confuses them. It's their response to it.

► Low Self-Esteem

Maybe the single most common characteristic among people with ADD is low self-esteem. With a past of endless failure, projects started and never finished, and being constantly at odds with their parents, siblings, teachers, and bosses, they tend to think of themselves as bad characters, deficient, aimless, lazy— embracing the terms and characterizations others use to describe them. After all, if a fish is sent to flying school and fails wing training, it's likely to feel bad about itself. So too, people who are ADD are constantly failing what doesn't fit.

► Rigidity

Right or wrong, people who are ADD seem inflexible, seem to lack finesse, and will pursue a course of action seemingly without regard to the consequences. Their sensitivity and anger can be like blinders, with their impulsiveness acting like a goad to drive them down a path to self-destruction. To them, it may be the rational, moral, survival action to take, but to us it appears reckless.

Consider the case of Lenny, just diagnosed with ADD and beginning therapy.

Lenny is 23, a college graduate, a bit of a hot-head, and turning into a very good salesman. He likes selling and liked his job until recently, when his old boss was transferred and a new one moved in.

The old boss was a kind, compassionate man who trusted Lenny, and if he had something to say to Lenny, he never sounded like he was criticizing him. And he extended generosity to other salespeople. Sales reports were normally due by two o'clock Friday, but the boss extended the deadline for one salesman, who always had lunch with his daughter on Friday. The salesman was divorced and missed his daughter very much, and lunching with her was important to him. Extending the report deadline for him was no problem for anyone.

When the new boss came on board, it was another story. The man was a critical, toe-the-line kind of guy who raised his voice whether he needed to or not and felt obligated to point out that he was boss. Even before he got to know anyone, he started handing out orders. Reports—all reports—had to be in by two o'clock Friday. When the salesman who had lunch with his daughter politely asked for an extension of one hour, explaining the circumstances, the new boss gruffly replied "No extensions, no exceptions. A job is a job and if you can't do it, I'll find someone who can."

All the other salespeople in the office glanced at each other but stayed quiet, burying their heads in their work. But Lenny, who already felt annoyed by the sound of the man's voice and attitude, couldn't stand it. It wasn't fair to his friend. No one else cared if the salesman's report was in by two o'clock.

Lenny got up and walked over to the new boss and right in front of everyone said, with raised voice, "That's not right. You shouldn't have done that. He's a good worker and it doesn't hurt anyone to extend his deadline. You have no right to do it."

The boss yelled "Sit down!" and Lenny stalked out of the office yelling "You're crazy. You've got no right to come in here and treat people that way."

When a friend tried to talk to him later, he was still hot under the collar and refused to apologize or back off. In fact, he quit the next day when, upon returning to pick up his worksheet for the day, he ran into his boss, who demanded an apology and started to lecture him. Lenny exploded and walked out, trapped by his ADD.

▶ Another Brand of Pain

I met Cynthia one evening at a middle-school parents' meeting. Disturbed and distracted by the chaotic approach to the session, my mind wandered over the day's events and my feet fidgeted. Cynthia, in contrast, looked so serene, unruffled by the politics of the organization and the lack of orderliness to the evening's agenda.

As I came to know Cynthia better, I came to understand that her quiet passivity was a cover for the wholesale confusion of ADD.

In reality, Cynthia was the over-controlled, passive type of ADD adult. She had crawled far inside herself, away from the world around her. It was the only way she could cope with the pain of ADD.

And, she had so restricted her environment that her ADD simply didn't show except when you got to know her intimately. All the symptoms were there. Her newsletters were always late, and, though she had a terrible struggle getting them together, she would accept no help. Not out of obstinacy or self-reliance, but out of shame. She didn't want anyone to see her work habits—which were like a page out of science fiction. Her home, too, was total chaos.

Cynthia's sense of competence was very low, which made her

feel that she didn't quite belong. But she covered her discomfort by seeming a bit of a know-it-all at times, which put others off.

Her way of coping with ADD had shaped her personality, if not robbed her of it, for she had, in fact, sacrificed her personality at the altar of ADD.

Adults with ADD feel angry, frustrated, confused, and out of control. They can be chronically depressed—stuck in their grief, but grief over what they don't know. Their fear of failure—as Cynthia shows us—is enormous and repressive. And no wonder, when we consider how their lives have been filled with failure. Why *would* anyone so used to failure want to undertake new experiences or entire new situations that seem to set them up for yet more failure?

Where most of us feel moments of low self-esteem, the ADD person feels it all the time; it is a permanent state of being, and it causes him or her great pain.

Such is the living hell of the ADD person.

◄ ı ◄ ı ◄ ı 5 ı ► ı ► ı ►

Living with an ADD Person

▼

*H*aving ADD is terribly painful, but living with an ADD person presents a whole new set of problems. Consider this letter from the wife of a man with ADD:

"Jack seemed like such a nice guy—agreeable, bright, well read, well educated and creative. His potential seemed enormous. He had big dreams and seemed to have all the skills needed to accomplish the task at hand—only he rarely did.

"He worked a lot, don't get me wrong, but he somehow failed to get ahead as far as it seemed that he could or should. It frustrated him, and the more frustrated he became, the more he pulled into himself. He began to appear more of a taker than a giver—a bottomless pit. Rarely did he get it together enough to give back.

"Resentment at his not giving back became my major emotion—and resentment on Jack's part grew as my expectations pressed him. He wasn't getting enough out of his own life to have anything left over for anyone else.

"I know now, after the divorce, that he is ADD, and that he didn't have anything left to give. But I didn't know that then. Not that he was mean or anything like that. Jack didn't blow up. He just withdrew, spending large amounts of time watching movies and television. Though he didn't exactly seem lazy (since he was willing enough to go out and earn a living) he seemed to have no time for household chores, self-care, or quiet conversation. In fact, he often fell asleep as soon as he sat down in the evenings.

"His social skills seemed flawed. Some of that had to do with the give-and-take required of socializing, but there was something more. He didn't plan ahead, often acted impulsively, and seemed unable to orchestrate spontaneous enterprises so they would come off successfully.

"I'll give you an example, one that happened after the divorce. Our son had an out-of-town football game and Jack offered to pick up me after work for the hour-long drive. The invitation came the afternoon of the game. I remembered the problems from the past, how he had trouble getting places on time. But I said 'Fine,' and added 'It's very important to me to get there for the start of the game.' Jack agreed.

"The game began at 7:30 PM. I suggested we set out at 5:30 so there would be time to grab a bite to eat. He said, 'Okay.' Then he arrived at six o'clock. But there was still plenty of time. As we headed down the freeway, he suddenly exited. 'Where are you going?' I asked. 'Home to change clothes,' Jack said.

"Again I said, 'Jack, it's very important to me to get to the game on time.'

"'I know,' he said.

"Jack changed quickly enough so that we still had time to go to a fast-food place. But, leaving his apartment, he started to turn right at the corner rather than go back to the freeway. When I asked where he was going, he said 'to get chicken' and named a restaurant several miles out of the way. I remembered how fussy Jack was about his food and how picking a place to eat could become a major stumbling block to peace.

But getting to the game on time was a higher priority, so I said, 'That'll take too long. Let's go on. Maybe we'll find a chicken place in the town.'

"If my response seems like incredible forbearance, it wasn't. In the old days, I'd have been boiling with frustration, anxiety, and disappointment. But, by now, I realized that Jack wasn't trying to be difficult. Nor was he trying to be mean. He just seemed unable to be aware of my needs even though—through therapy—I'd learned to speak them clearly. Just like always, he was getting off the track he'd agreed to. I used to think it was because he agreed to things he didn't want. Or that he was being resistant to me on purpose. But, after I came to understand ADD, I realized it was neither. He just didn't get things done efficiently.

"We arrived at the town sooner than expected and cruised around because he wanted to see what restaurants there were to choose from. I wanted to stop at the first place we found just so we could get to the game on time. But that wouldn't do for Jack. His feelings of being cheated, something that grew out of his ADD, often had spilled over into other areas, and he was fussy about buying anything. What made him a good shopper in other situations was maddening in this one.

"Finally, we got back to the first place we'd seen and I nudged him into accepting it. Though we ordered our food to go, he without thinking, ordered something that was complicated to get together. With kickoff time fast approaching, he leisurely added salad bar toppings to his food and, then, midstream, became distracted by the potato bar. As I watched, I realized he wasn't being mean. He just couldn't help it. But I remember why I'd divorced him and reminded myself to drive my own car next time there was an out-of-town game. We were late to the game. Shades of an angry, frustrating past."

Those who live with an untreated, unrecognized ADD person are very often victims as well. Whether the keynote to the ADD personality is flaring temper, unpredictability, chemical addiction, or constant disorganization, the behavior can be extremely difficult to cope with, even for caring and sensitive people. Unaware of ADD, parents, spouses, and siblings can become resentful and angry; they can feel exploited, disappointed, or cheated. None of these feelings make for healthy relationships.

▶ The Frustration

One teenager summed up how it was to live with his ADD brother: "It's frustrating."

Yes, that's a normal response to any sibling, but it's the ways in which the frustration comes out that makes the difference. I think the difference is in the "sharp corners" of an ADD personality. It's the abrasiveness that is so often present in relationships with an ADD person. It's their immediate "No" to most requests.

One brother mentioned how his ADD brother was prone to be combative. A mild pop on the arm became a "federal case" and was likely to be turned into a fight—maybe good-humored—but not one the ADD person could ever walk away from or be the first to stop. This included love pats that were interpreted as assaults instead of gestures of friendship. Sensitivity in action!

Another sibling—a sister—talked about how her ADD sister tended to pick fights "out of thin air." Her view was representative of many others who noted in their siblings with ADD a tendency to make things happen when everything was quiet. Almost as if boredom threatened them, they seem to kick up dust for interest's sake.

▶ The Nuisance

The word "nuisance" also comes up frequently along with examples of attention-getting behavior. If five people are in a group, and one is ADD, that is the person who will unwittingly but most likely draw attention to himself.

Because they draw attention so easily, it's very easy for children to set up their brother or sister with ADD in the good guy/bad guy syndrome. Of course, any healthy sibling will jump at a chance to fight back in an argument, or at least gain brownie points with parents at the expense of the sibling. But when the sibling has ADD, it's not a fair contest.

▶ Don't Touch Me

Intimacy, so wonderful an experience for most of us, is often denied the people who live with an ADD person. For intimacy is a major challenge—if not an impossibility—for an ADD person.

They seem to feel everything excessively, from innuendoes to touch. As babies, ADD persons are extremely sensitive. The normal things—rocking, holding, stroking—that a parent may do to soothe a baby don't work with an ADD baby. It upsets him. Thus, with no awareness of ADD, the parent may feel rejected by the baby, and intimacy is destroyed. Even as the child grows, his sensitivity to touch is unabated. Parents—and siblings—may be denied the familiarity of throwing a friendly arm around a shoulder.

And they may encounter a wall of distrust that goes beyond the physical. The person with ADD, battered by an unrelenting environment, may seek safety inside, withdrawing indiscriminately from friend and foe alike.

It's not just the ADD person's hypersensitivity that inhibits intimacy. Remember, they tend to be full on or full off. They can come home, plop down in front of the television, and be fast asleep in a couple of minutes. There is no chance for the development that leads to intimacy.

Sex with an ADD spouse can be something out of the one-minute manager's handbook. Frustrating? A nuisance? Destructive? You pick it.

▶ Who's To Blame?

The ADD person is almost obsessive about blame, for blame is the major perspective from which his life is structured. Some of this occurs, no doubt, from being chided for nonconstructive behaviors in early life. Persons with ADD live with blame. They learn blame as a way of life. Also, it's simpler to take a frustrating experience and blame it on someone or something than to think through why and how things happen. Very likely the intensity of feeling experienced by the ADD person requires a short-circuited, quick resolution to the pain—and blame provides that. Besides, if the way you're wired is considered unacceptable from day one of your life, you are likely to use any opportunity to fend off the hurt.

But for those living with the ADD person, his need to blame is often experienced as hostile needless—and painful—behavior. Most relationships are damaged by the placement of blame. It's no way to build trust, the glue of all relationships, and it sets a win-lose thinking in operation. It seems that the ADD person's finger is always pointed at those he lives with.

▶ The Damage

In practical terms, what all this boils down to for parents, spouses, siblings, and even friends is a wearing, tearing, thorn-in-the-side relationship.

Brothers and sisters see the ADD person's short attention span as a nuisance that gets in the way of peaceful, stable play activities. They see their ADD sibling getting in trouble a lot and often fall into the good kid/bad kid routine. The ADD children don't take orders well and tend to cause explosive situations. Their brothers and sisters who are non-ADD don't understand the disruption.

Mom and Dad tend to spend more time with the ADD child, though that time usually isn't constructive—so parents often get used to interacting with the child as a problem child. This can make parents feel guilty. I doubt there's a parent of an untreated ADD child who hasn't asked "Where did I go wrong? What have I done?"

Face it: Living or working with a person with untreated, undiagnosed ADD can be an angry, frustrating experience, full of disappointment, resentment, and dissatisfaction for all.

◄ ◄ ◄ 6 ► ► ►

The Quandary
of Treatment

▼

S herry originally came into therapy wanting help with her second marriage. She was angry at her husband because he didn't take enough financial responsibility, and the children (his and hers) were erupting right and left. There were personal motivations, too. Her mood swings, evident all her life, seemed to be growing more extreme. Her ability to focus on a task and complete it seemed to have diminished rather than grown.

But she seemed eager to get things right in her life, ready to work at therapy. The only problem to the upbeat beginning was that Sherry had a different agenda every time she came in for therapy. Every time she agreed to work on an issue, something got in the way and follow-through was avoided. She would go off in a dozen directions the minute she walked out of my office.

Sherry's husband, though not as scattered, was no better than she was at follow-through. He made even bigger promises that he didn't keep. Working with the two of them was next to impossible.

Going through problems with each of their five children as the teenage years came on had left Sherry and her husband no bet-

51

ter able to take charge. They knew what to do, it seemed, but couldn't accomplish it.

Then the husband's financial irresponsibility left them in a lot of trouble which Sherry felt helpless to remedy. And Sherry, who for years had worked with her father (a drinker who had encouraged dependence in Sherry) was left without a job when he retired; the secure, if damaging, daily routine that had put structure in her life was eliminated.

Her husband's response was to face the music (his accountant and the IRS) and clean up his act. He stopped drinking, shaped up physically, and began to take responsibility in his business.

But is wasn't long after that that Sherry began drinking heavily and abusing her body in other ways—binging on caffeine products and eating and sleeping erratically. Other self-destructive behavior began to emerge. Sherry began to act out her feelings which meant, in her words, "pulling a runaway." She'd simply leave home, taking up with whomever she met. Maybe she'd have an affair; maybe just a friendship punctuated by emotional highs.

She'd claim great insights into her psychology from these episodes, but her scattered behavior didn't change, nor did her life smooth out. Much of the acting out was met with passivity by her husband, while her father supplied financial support so that Sherry could remain irresponsible. She continued being out of control for almost two years until she became an excessive financial liability and her mood swings (days spent in bed) had increased to the point where they could no longer be ignored. She was hospitalized four times during the next year.

Professionals who worked with Sherry disagreed about what was wrong with her. Their diagnoses ranged from alcoholism to Attention Deficit Disorder, manic-depression characterized by wide mood swings, and borderline personality characterized by a pervasive pattern of instability, with a few others thrown in for good measure.

Maybe they were all correct, for Sherry was a classic example of a person displaying multiple disorders, or at least the symptoms of such. Her childhood history—at school and in the family—indicated that she certainly was ADD. She was a member of a dysfunctional family riddled by addiction and codependency. Sherry never properly separated from her family of origin (parents) to become an independent person with value in her own right. She lived at a survival level most of the time, just barely able to show enough responsibility to get by. Her biochemistry was out of balance, in part because she did not attend to her nutrition, exercise, and rest. Her mood swings, from extreme emotional highs to severe depression, were separated by periods of normal mood.

An extreme case? You bet, but Sherry's situation points up how difficult it can be to make a proper ADD diagnosis when other disorders may be present and symptoms may overlap. ADD is basic neurobiochemical brainwiring that underlies or coexists with other physiology and learned behavior. It's not a "diagnosis" of exclusion any more than skin color. Organizational problems may be a sign of other learning disabilities. Mood variability can be the result of hormones, nutritional inadequacies, and stress. Impulsivity and overreactivity can be the result of poor or inadequate training or other organic difficulties, including seizure disorders.

To further complicate the problem, mimicking symptoms may be present: Stress and emotional difficulties can mock many ADD symptoms such as inattentiveness, mood swings, low self-esteem, and anger.

Is it any wonder that a definitive diagnosis can be difficult? Though sorting through the look-alike symptoms is confusing, it's important to try not to boil a person's behavior and make-up down to one label.

▶ What about Medication?

Once a person is formally labeled as ADD, the next step raises an argument among professionals. Some want to treat ADD so the person can approximate normalcy. Some use medication and other training procedures that make ADD people more like non-ADD people. And some, like myself, want to train and educate people who are ADD to use their natural skills effectively and learn other skills that are not natural, so that they can fit into a non-ADD culture while maintaining self-esteem and their unique individuality.

Use of medication is common in ADD children, but, in ADD adults, its use is erratic, inconsistent, and, frankly, confusing even from the professional's point of view. Raise the question of medicating ADD adults in a group of mental health workers and you'll see the fur fly. I am neither for nor against medication. But a person must understand its use is to help someone fit into a setting that is not natural, such as to sit at a desk for long periods of time doing paperwork that is required by a job.

I have heard contradictory statistical claims about the use of medication with adults, from "it never works" to "it works sixty percent of the time." Many ADD people initially have gained unexpected relief from their ADD symptoms when they used diet pills. They became, as one person put it, "instantly mature and responsible." Unfortunately, the relief lasts only as long as the supply of diet pills. Then they revert back to their old, familiar ADD behavior.

There is strong resistance to the use of the drug Ritalin. I have been told that, though commonly used in childhood ADD, it is *never* appropriate with adults. Yet I've seen many people whose lives have been transformed because of its use. My own son did not reap the full benefits of nine months of counseling, which he received at age eleven, until he started taking Ritalin at thirteen. It helped him control his actions with less than gargantuan effort. Once on medication, he almost instantly showed the effects of counseling and could get himself to do what he really wanted to do all along. He never did want to be disruptive in groups or insensitive to the needs of others; he simply couldn't sit still or keep his mouth shut. Once the medication allowed the therapy to take hold, however, he could show that he really was sensitive to others' needs. It also bought him time to learn the behaviors expected by the settings in which he found himself. Then he was able to discontinue its use for behavioral reasons and only use it when doing sustained paperwork.

I promise you, I have no vested interest in any particular drug being prescribed. But what does interest me is the strong reaction against it, unsubstantiated by research. As one physician put it, prescribing Ritalin "is just never done." Yet another practitioner I ran into was as extreme but in the opposite direction, diagnosing ADD willy-nilly in his patients—and treating them all with Ritalin.

Antidepressants, on the other hand, are sometimes tried first as an adult ADD treatment—for those physicians who believe in the condition at all. In fact, several physicians I've run across not only preferred their use in treatment, but continued to prescribe their use whether they were effective or not on the patient's ADD. Frequently, stimulants such as Ritalin, antidepressants, or other medications are used simultaneously with considerable effectiveness. However, physicians cannot tell which drug or combination of drugs will work with which people, nor the amount required for effectiveness.

Another point of debate has been drug treatment of ADD chemical abusers. Many chemically dependent ADD people are successfully treated with ADD medications. The individual must, however, acknowledge a problem with chemical abuse and be abstaining from chemical usage. Then treatment with medication for ADD is appropriate.

Remember, though, medication must never be the only intervention for ADD. Alone it is inadequate to treat ADD. Training and education must accompany drug therapy to teach the skills needed to manage ADD. Simultaneously, finding the environment that fits a person with ADD wiring must happen. There are no magic changes, but learning to both accommodate and utilize your ADD effectively is possible.

► Therapy?

There has been little precedent for the "treatment" of Attention Deficit Disorder in adults. Remember, clinicians have long been polarized on the question of whether ADD in adults is a reality. When this book was originally published, many were unwilling to look openly at the possibility that it exists. Indeed, beginning in the late 1970s, the bible of the American Psychiatric Association, the *Diagnostic Statistical Manual of Mental Disorders* designated ADD-RT as a viable diagnosis when Attention Deficit Disorder continued into adulthood. But when the DSM III-R came out in 1987, ADD-RT was eliminated. In its place was a listing of Undifferentiated ADD, with a note that research is necessary to determine if this is a valid diagnostic category and, if so, how it should be defined. We've come a long way since.

Just as challenging for the professional community has been arriving at a consensus on how to counsel ADD adults. First of all, there has been little therapy, counseling, teaching, or guidance of any kind available for ADD adults. Second, people with ADD tend to be quite creative. Though they need structure, they also need to be involved in developing their own structure so that they can carry it out independently. Thus, traditional psychotherapy often doesn't work, and the results of such attempts are often very uneven as the following case indicates:

A woman who had been in treatment for almost two years continued to cut deals with her husband, agreeing to be more conscientious about running the house and managing the affairs of everyday life. She and her therapist had determined that she really wanted these goals and intended to follow through. They had examined unconscious motives and childhood-connected reasons why she couldn't—or didn't—follow through. They had looked at the marriage with the concomitant issues of control and power and discovered that these issues were in balance. In short, they covered every conventional base. Why, then, didn't the woman respond to the conventional therapy? You guessed it!

A bright business executive with a technical background repeatedly suffered emotional stress at work because he failed to guide the people who worked under him through the complex projects they were assigned. He could do the technical part in his head but became overwhelmed and lost with the myriad details that management requires. He would become irritable and gripe at his people, and morale would plummet. His home life, never smooth, suffered when "one more thing requiring management" was necessary.

He was in individual psychotherapy as well as marriage counseling but continued to perform in dysfunctional ways. He also became quite depressed as the counseling proved ineffective and was treated with antidepressants. They didn't do any good, either.

There are other dangers in therapy. One therapist I know of accurately diagnosed ADD in his clients but treated them in a manner similar to that used with people in denial who suffer from chemical abuse problems. He pressured his clients into following a rigid structure he had developed. This approach, however, only kept clients coming to him for years because they remained dependent, helplessly trying to fit into his structure. Often their depression continued because they could not become independent of the therapist.

These are not uncommon instances; rather, they are common, and point out popular misconceptions and mistreatment in counseling persons with ADD, including:

▶ Regarding ADD as an emotional disorder rather than a physiologically based style of brain wiring that affects behavior and learning styles.

▶ Misdiagnosis that results in treatment of childhood and parenting causes, behind which is the belief that ADD is the result of poor parenting or a dysfunctional family system.

► A belief that ADD people can control their behavior if they just want to. (This leads the therapist to focus on why people with ADD don't want to control their behavior.)

► Using insight therapy—training the ADD person in life skills rather than teaching the person how to recognize and accommodate the ADD.

► Failing to treat ADD after chemical abuse is stemmed.

► Marriage counseling that doesn't recognize the existence of ADD.

► Therapy that allows the therapist's own beliefs and prejudices about ADD to interfere with counseling.

Such is the quandary of ADD treatment.

► Some Common Questions on the Treatment of ADD

► Will I become a zombie on medication?

Absolutely not, if the kind and dosage is properly prescribed. Medications for Attention Deficit Disorder help a person to be able to do tasks that are not natural. It helps them "fit in" better to a non-ADD culture.

► How can I find a therapist who can help me learn to live with my ADD?

Unfortunately, that is not an easy task because very few psychotherapists, counselors, or educators have had training in working with adults who have ADD. Try locally first, checking with your Mental Health Association to see whether there is a support group established in your area. They will have a list of people who regularly work with ADD. If you have no luck, contact one of the national organizations listed at the end of this book.

▶ **How can I find a doctor who could prescribe medication if it is indicated?**

Again, try through your local support group. Ask your physician if he or she is knowledgeable about ADD or would be willing to learn.

▶ **Why does ADD show up so often after chemical abuse is treated? Does the chemical abuse cause ADD?**

No. If, indeed, ADD appears after a person has "dried out," it would have been there all along but simply wasn't visible. One of the reasons is that untreated people with ADD are prone to self-medicate and one of the ways to do that is with alcohol or drugs. People who are ADD are also prone to impulsive behavior and may more readily be swept along with the crowd, succumbing to peer pressure and thus establishing a chemical habit.

It is important that an accurate diagnosis of ADD be made after chemical abuse has taken place because attention problems are prevalent for other reasons for a period of time after sobriety is achieved.

▶ **Is ADD always present after chemical abuse is controlled?**

No. Only some chemical abusers will show ADD brain wiring. But more and more people with chemical abuse problems are being identified as ADD.

◄ ı ◄ ı ◄ | 7 |► ı► ı ►

The Way Out

▼

*T*here is a way out of ADD. But, remember, you won't "cure" it. You don't want to eliminate it, for it is the basic way your brain is wired and there's nothing "wrong" with it.

What you can do is manage it. My style of therapeutic intervention—which I developed through counseling hundreds of ADD persons—is actually a mixture of education, training, and therapy that recognizes the potential assets of ADD and the harm it has caused.

This calls for identifying ADD and accepting that you are the way your are, working through and correcting the damage it has caused, and restructuring your life to accommodate it. Don't be ashamed of it. Face it, you probably didn't even know you had it.

► The Diagnosis

The first step is identification. I have discovered that people with ADD, once alerted to ADD's possible existence, are quite good at self-diagnosis. (If you are the least bit hesitant to undertake the task yourself, find a therapist who acknowledges the existence of adult ADD and enlist his help.)

The identification must include a thorough childhood history. Preferably work it up with a parent, sibling, other family member, or childhood friend; they can be a marvelous aid in helping you get outside yourself and see your life from a totally different perspective.

School performance is a frequent indicator of ADD. Phrases are a dead giveaway: "If only he'd pay attention . . . ," "She's so bright, but she just doesn't finish her work," "His mind keeps wandering," or "She fidgets and wastes time."

The level of family peace often reflects the presence of an ADD child. When the ADD child was absent, things often ran more smoothly and with less turmoil. When the ADD child reappeared, disruption and chaos were not far behind—not in an ugly way, just in a frazzled way. Disciplinary and guidance methods had to be changed. Generally, more time was spent paying attention to the ADD child and more intercession with the world outside the family was necessary. Parents often were required to help the ADD child get along with friends and siblings. Memories of many fights and conflicts, uncompleted chores, and time spent focused on an overreactive son or daughter can be indicators of ADD. Many ADD children, because of their impulsivity, may have had more accidents than other children in the family. Try to recall how often the child was heard saying "I'm sorry." He really didn't mean to do wrong. He just did it. And, as though he failed to learn from experience, his childhood is likely to have been filled with repeat offenses. If you are a parent and suspect that your grown child has ADD, you may have felt that, as a child, he or she was out to get you.

In addition to an inventory of childhood history, it is also helpful to inventory a checklist of typical ADD behaviors in adults. (If you suspect that you have ADD, it will be useful to go over this list with someone close to you, because you may be unaware of your own behaviors.):

Inattention: Often fails to finish things started; often does not seem to listen; easily distracted; difficulty concentrating on sustained-attention tasks; difficulty sticking to an activity.

Impulsivity: Often acts before thinking; shifts excessively from one activity to another; has difficulty working independently; frequently talks out or interrupts; finds it difficult to wait his turn.

Hyperactivity: Paces or moves a lot; has difficulty staying seated; moves about excessively during sleep; always on the go.

Emotionality: Very sensitive to rejection and frustration; shifts moods suddenly and unexpectedly; frequent negative thinking even about success or accomplishment (stemming from the belief that such success is impossible); unexplained chronic recurring depression; finds being soothed and held most difficult; needs excessive sensory input such as television or music to blot out extraneous noise.

It is useful to write down descriptive comments and anecdotes for each behavior or characteristic as you go through the assessment, and take them from both the present time and from childhood. They will help in determining the presence of ADD as well as in differentiating ADD from other conditions.

Finally, check your family history. Frequently a parent will have had ADD traits that went undiagnosed in earlier years. Sometimes it will be another family member from the previous generation. Remember, ADD tends to run in families.

▶ Self-Image

It is impossible to suffer from unrecognized ADD without some poor living habits building up. New training is necessary so the newly identified person with ADD isn't set up for failure. You can get beyond ADD, but it's imperative to make adjustments for your ADD so that its effects can be nullified. You must develop a new self-image and adjust to that new self-image—one in which you see yourself as okay.

Self-images build slowly and change just as slowly. Once we get used to one, it's a bit hard to let go of it. And it feels better to hang on to a poor self-image than to strive for a good self-image because of the fear of failing to live up to a good one. If many childhood incidents have proven over and over that you are a failure or, at best, an underachiever, then your willingness to risk will be limited.

So, I ask you to:

1) Assess how you are doing now and how you've been doing (you may want to use a scale of one to five where one equals poorly, three is okay, and five superlative);

2) Make a list of traits you'd like to leave behind you. Include particular traits that cost you a lot to continue to carry. Examples include temper (blowing up under stress), blaming (accusing others for problems rather than looking at your own part in things), quitting (running away from difficult situations), and procrastination. With all of these traits, you end up losing a lot of yourself even though you gain a sense of protection—at least temporarily. (Each behavior represents a psychological attempt to protect your vulnerable feelings.)

3) Make a list of traits that you'd like to have or that you admire in others.

4) Adopt those traits. If some are made difficult by ADD, such as staying on task, commit to doing what you can do about it. Team up with others to help you. Then drop responsibility for what you can't do. Take small steps.

5) Look at your new identity as someone who is ADD and is working with it. Embrace it as your own. Say good-bye to the old and reach out for the new.

And when it comes to self-image, remember, too, that being ADD is not all bad. Being a poor robot or assembly line worker means you have more time to be creative. You see the world a little bit differently than others. These are special gifts. Explore them. Just because people in this culture believe there is a right way—the non-ADD way—of doing things does not mean your way is wrong. Our culture just has trouble honoring differences. Exercise your way of doing things. It's important for you to develop approaches and methods that make you feel competent.

For example, a lot is made about leaving assignments to the last minute. But does it really matter? Our culture is into planning early, but does it really matter when an assignment is started? No! It just needs to get done. And working one hour each day for five days is no "better" than working five hours in one day, even if it's the last day.

So, why not give yourself permission to start late and enjoy the doing—as long as it's done on time—instead of punishing yourself with scoldings?

Enjoy your individuality. Feel good about what you are instead of worrying about what you're not. You are you, and there is no one who's better at being that.

▶ The Group Effect

When ADD has gone unrecognized in childhood, the initial reaction in the adult—after diagnosis—is relief; relief at finding an explanation for much of what has caused disruption and unfulfilled potential in the person's life. Euphoria may accompany the relief. Whew! It feels as if anything is possible.

At this point, it is good to talk with others about the awareness of ADD. The discussion helps ground the person until there is time to catch up with the new identity.

Most communities will have a self-help clearinghouse and a guide to local services. The Mental Health Association is a good place to start. Also, schools will have contacts for parents of children with ADD. In turn, they may know whether there is an adult group. Find one of these groups and join. If no group is available locally, form your own. (See appendices for more information.)

Talk about your feelings with others in the group. First talk openly about your feelings of having a lifelong condition. Begin to connect with others in the group, people who have the same characteristics you have. Realize you share a common bond with people who have the same kinds of problems with attention you have. Realize that you all are sensitive, probably very creative, and abused to varying degrees, depending on how well your ways were understood and tolerated as a child. Each of you will share a characteristic way of reacting to the world, and it feels really good to know that you're not alone.

Sharing experiences with the group will be quite helpful. For example, you might tell the group, "At noon, my wife asked me to mow the lawn, and I said I'd do it before she got back from the beauty shop. As she left, she mentioned she'd like to go to the movies that evening, and I said, okay. But then I spotted last week's mail on the desk, so I began to go through it. I knew she got mad when I didn't get to it in a timely manner. Then I got hungry and decided to go the grocery store. On the way home I saw my friend, Sam. We talked and he made me remember I'd never returned the books to the library. I figured I'd better do it because she gets mad when I don't. I was just ready to get the mower out when my wife got home. Furiously, she told me I'd ruined her evening. She'd really wanted to go to the movies. She's always blowing up. And I'm always goofing up."

Now, in order to understand the situation, the group might do a feelings analysis. Note how each person felt, starting with you. You might say something like, "I felt fine all afternoon. I thought I was doing what my wife likes. I had a good time and was glad to see an old friend. I was glad to see my wife and didn't mean to hurt her."

Than you would analyze your wife's feelings: "She seemed to leave in a happy mood. She even seemed happy when she first drove in the driveway, but then immediately got mad."

Now you might ask your group members to help you figure out what happened and how you can manage things better in the future.

Basically, you committed to mowing the lawn by the time your wife got home, but you didn't. And you led her to believe you'd go to a movie. From her perspective, she thought she had an agreement that would lead to the lawn being done and an entertaining evening at the movies. If you didn't want to go and had said so, she could have gotten a friend to go with her, if it was important to her.

You, in turn, meant no harm. You tried to do too much to please her and didn't plan your time well. And you really want to be a nice guy, so lots of times you agree to things you're not very crazy about doing. And then it's even easier for you to get off track. And you also said "uh-huh" to your wife about the movies, perhaps wanting to please her, but forgetting you have to make such things happen. Or maybe, with the "uh-huh," you were just affirming her existence without really listening to the content of her request.

Your group will care about you. Use them to learn new ways. Learn to see yourself as you are and work to change what you don't like.

▶ Use the Word "No"

Above all, stop being the good guy unless you really are willing to take responsibility to follow through. It's not so bad to say "no." It's a lot easier on those around you. They may even respect you more.

If, by chance, you run into someone who won't take no for an answer, just turn the responsibility over to them, saying "I don't mean to hurt or frustrate you, but I'm not going to commit to something I may not follow through on." The other person may not like it, if that person is overly dependent on you to get his or her needs met, but you can't be responsible for that anyway, so stick to your guns. Learn to say "No!"

Use your group's help by making a commitment to say "no." Report back each week on how well you've done this and count on positive reinforcement from people who care and understand.

► Common Questions about Getting Help

► Why do people with ADD so often have negative thinking after an accomplishment?

For one thing, most ADD people have learned to think of themselves as inadequate. They tend to have developed low self-esteem which makes them think of all kinds of reasons why what they did couldn't possibly have come because of the capability.

Also, their negative thinking serves as a protection against someone else saying something negative first.

► With the extra sensitivity that ADD people have, how can working with a radio or TV on help them concentrate?

It serves as a kind of white noise, a constant sound, that masks discrepant or irregular sounds or sights that they would experience as more disruptive. Also there is a consistent rhythm or sameness to TV and radio sounds. (The technical directors of the stations make sure that this is true, I promise you.) The consistency soothes an ADD person.

► Does the use of medication diminish the positive traits of an ADD person, such as creativity or the ability to synthesize information and make unusual connections?

Probably not. It does help the person focus more constructively on the expression of those traits. Check for
yourself.

► **Can an ADD person juggle lots of things at the same
time?**

Often. In fact, it may help them to get things done to
have several things going at one time so that they have a
reason to move from one thing to another and a specific
place to put their attention when they get bored with
the original activity. This keeps them from going off
willy-nilly.

► **In addition to being creative, are there other positive
traits of ADD and does it take having ADD to have
them?**

Traits, such as creativity and the lack of boundary isolation that leads to cross disciplinary tendencies are
only the beginning of the positive uses for the sensitivity created by ADD. In addition, there are interpersonal
ones; empathy, sensitivity to others, the ability to see
through facades and view people and situations as
they really are, and an openness to sharing thoughts
and feelings.

These traits are, of course, shared by others who do not
have ADD. But the existence of ADD gives people a
built in head start.

► **Why would a person who finds out he has ADD feel
"as if anything is possible"?**

For one thing, it's like popping the cork on a bottle of
champagne. It flies high from having been under pressure. The awareness of what his problem is opens new
doorways previously closed. The ADD person has no
experience in the new "world" by which to gauge limits.

69

Time and experience will define some limits, but initially it seems that the sky's the limit.

► **Why would you have to teach a person with ADD to say "No," when you stated earlier that persons with ADD often say it automatically?**

Initially people with ADD say "no" as a way of buying time and power. "No" pushes the person with the request away and puts the control in the hands of the person who has ADD. Since people with ADD tend to feel intruded upon, they need such a barrier for protection.

Later, as people with ADD become socialized, they learn to be "nice guys" in order to get approval and tend to say "yes" automatically in order to please. A person with ADD needs to learn to stop and think whether he really wants to do something or is just trying to please or to get the person with the request off his back without making a fuss.

Saying "no" without thinking is non-constructive. Saying "no" with thought is constructive.

► **Sometimes my attention is better than at other times. What can I do to help myself?**

First, be kind and understanding to yourself. Be sure you're doing something that fits you.

Next, check to see what things may be interfering with your attention: nutrition, tiredness, stress. Ask yourself whether you have disrupted your usual schedule in any area.

Correct the disruption. Consistent structure in your life is your best friend.

▶ **What can I do to get myself to finish things I start?**

Be sure you are trying to do something that is important to you.

Give yourself an incentive to work for, promising yourself that you'll treat yourself when you complete the task. Be sure to break whatever you're doing into manageable segments and give yourself breaks along the way. But time your breaks so you keep them under control.

◄ ◄ ◄ 8 ► ► ►

The Visualization
Technique

▼

*T*here are those of you reading
this book whose pain is indeed great from your growing-up
years. Hurt, abuse, and anger—and more hurt—were so mon-
umental you couldn't escape them, let alone do anything
about them. Remember, abuse from ADD may have resulted
from benign circumstances, but nonetheless it was there. A
legacy remains from teachers, parents, and employers whose
personal goals—to train you properly—were thwarted by
your being ADD and who became frustrated. The abuse may
have come in the form of well-meant scoldings or behavioral
limits that you couldn't abide, such as groundings or keeping
you after school. Of course, at times the abuse may have been
much more than that, including overreactive responses such
as actual physical punishment.

For you I want to suggest that you practice a technique used in
many fields for many purposes: visualization. I have, in dealing
with adults identified with ADD, made modifications in the
technique that make it both appropriate and successful for ADD
treatment. Look at it as a tool for "reparenting" yourself.

In a quiet place, sit in a comfortable chair that has arms, close
your eyes, and take a step back from your experience. Think of

something that makes you feel secure, very secure, safe, and protected. It might be sitting in the lap of your grandmother. Or it might be feeling the sun on your shoulder while you walk through a forest filled with the smell of springtime, a soft breeze against your cheek. Choose your own brand of safety—and feel the arm of the chair.

Imagine projecting your experience onto a movie screen, and view it as you might a movie. As you do this, grasp the arm of the chair that you're sitting in while watching the movie, and feel the security of it. You can even see yourself watching the movie.

(If you feel resistant to doing this exercise, don't do it. Your psyche is telling you: "Whoa, this is not good for me." You may wish to do this work with a counselor or not at all. Your psyche knows best; trust it.)

Now, let's all get ready to change history.

Let your mind drift back to a time in your youth when you felt misunderstood, inadequate, out of control. Visualize that part of you in your mind's eye. You will probably feel a sensation within you that reflects how you felt at the time. Pay particular attention to that feeling, its shape, its location in your physical body, and its size and substance. Is it hot or cold, hard or soft, solid or porous? Attach a color to it.

Immediately after defining it, squeeze the arm of the chair and find that nice, warm secure feeling. As you neutralize the sensation that causes you discomfort, realize that you can grow beyond your history.

Remember, if you are projecting this experience on a movie screen, keep it there while you watch yourself sitting and watching the movie.

Next, let your mind drift back to an earlier time in your life when you encountered a similar feeling. Locate its presence in your body again and visualize where you were standing as a child when it happened. What were you doing? Squeeze the arm of the chair. Remember to keep the vision on your movie screen.

Now, go back and seek the earliest experience you can recall when the same constellation of events or feelings took place. You may have been four, five, or six years old. Once more, squeeze the arm of the chair and check your movie screen if you need to.

It is now time to rewrite history.

Pretend you are a script writer. You have the capability to rewrite your childhood history any way you want. You can give your child words and understanding that realistically he or she would not have had. In this rewriting job, anything is possible. Also allow the others in your drama to have words, skills, and understanding they didn't actually have but that you can give them since you are recreating their characters.

Visualize the child with the out-of-control, inadequate feelings and let the child say what he or she needs: Understanding? Support? A sense of control? Your child might say something like: "I feel overwhelmed. I need you to understand that I'm trying as hard as I can." Squeeze the arm of the chair you're sitting in. Feel it holding you up.

Visualize the grownups in the child's life reassuring the child, giving him understanding, knowledge, whatever was needed. Hear them teaching the child: "You are ADD. It's no big deal. I can help you learn to overcome its effects. You are smart. You are okay. I love you. I'm here with you and I'll help you learn to pay attention. See, you are already doing it. You're a fast learner. I love you."

If you like, feel the warm arm of the adult around the child's shoulders. Watch the adult walk the child into school and explain to the teachers what is needed. See the teachers pass the message on. And see your child grow assured, secure, capable, and able to be in control.

If the adults in your early life were particularly abusive, see the child on the movie screen stop them. Have them freeze, like the child's game "Freeze," where no one can move without permission of the game leader. Let the child be the leader and call "freeze." Then let a special, understanding adult teach them about ADD.

Next, watch the abusive adults change their level of understanding, becoming enlightened. Let them say "I am so sorry. I didn't mean any harm. I didn't know any better. Please forgive me."

Watch the child on the screen take as long as he needs to do that. No rush. If the child needs to vent some anger, fine. If the child wants to scold, fine. When the feeling is vented and the child sees the adults for what they were—frightened, helpless, frustrated—forgiveness will come. But let it come in its own time as you again squeeze the arm of your chair, feeling the security it offers, the support and comfort.

Feel the child's growing sense of control. Realize that the feeling will spread and grow to be used daily as you go about your business in confidence, knowing that you are now understood and strong.

You can change each recalled experience this way. Give the child what is needed. Provide the child with the power of information and the support of understanding. Watch the child, adolescent, and adult in you grow in confidence before your mind's eye. Forgive those who hurt you out of ignorance and feel the confidence build within you to be in control of yourself as someone who is ADD. Simply make room for it when planning your activities.

► Dealing with Grief

In addition to the hurt and anger of abuse, you have to deal with the grief—over loss of potential—that ADD has brought into your life.

Remember that grief has several stages including denial, anger, bargaining, depression and acceptance. Remember, too, that you likely are stuck in some phase of the process of grieving and have never reached the acceptance stage. But you can.

Identify and vent your feelings. Acknowledge them to yourself—or at first just toy with the idea of them. Say them aloud to yourself and let yourself feel whatever you feel—depression, anger, denial. Then write down the feelings—and again let yourself feel whatever you feel.

Voice your feelings to someone else—a therapist, an understanding person, the group if you're in one—and let yourself feel whatever you feel. As the feelings wash through you, befriend the grieving part of you—the little boy who was so angry about feeling helpless, the young woman who felt so bad over being unable to keep the job she loved because she couldn't get the paperwork done on time.

Put your arm around the part of you that needs your help. When you have released the grief, raise your head, take a deep breath of fresh air, and get ready to develop new ways to reach your potential.

► Common Questions about Visualization

► What can I do if I can't get my mind to be quiet enough to do the visualization?

Make sure that you get into a regular daily habit of spending time quietly so that your mind and emotions can count on the time. Make a list of intruding concerns and problems that are most likely to distract you and commit to return to them at a later time. Slow your breathing down and feel it becoming a little deeper and more regular. Experiment to see which is easiest for you, closing your eyes, keeping your eyes open, or keeping your eyes open but focusing on one thing. Clear your mind further by letting a gentle breeze carry the thoughts off or take a mental broom and sweep them aside or place them on a shelf or in a box for later sorting.

Start the visualization but don't expect to finish it. Do it in stages, being easy on yourself.

► **What should I do if I start feeling very emotional during the visualization?**

Stop. Don't go further into it.

Allow yourself to stay with the feeling. Be gentle and nurturing with yourself. Express the feeling out loud to yourself, letting the adult part of you realize that your little kid part was deeply touched.

You may not want to do any further work with the visualization that day. You may want to talk with someone about the feelings. Do so. Return to the visualization at a time when it feels comfortable to do so.

► **What do I do if I have trouble seeing pictures in my mind or don't see them at all? Does that mean there is something else wrong with me?**

There is nothing wrong with you. Some people visualize easily. Other people are better at hearing dialogue in their heads. And still others do best feeling things.

If you are having trouble getting pictures in your mind,

try having a conversation with yourself and your inner child. Recall the conversations you had as a child, and remember what you heard that impressed you.

If this method still leaves you wanting, settle on feeling the experiences that you went through as a child and substitute the feeling you would have liked that child to have had. Bring the child feelings of joy and power. You can do this by recalling feelings of joy and power in other settings and transferring those feelings to your ADD experience.

▶ **When the history of my childhood is being rewritten, what do I do if I simply can't see my parents being helpful?**

Some people have to substitute other people for their parents. It may be an aunt or uncle, family friend, doctor, public figure, or someone from literature. Call forth the person you would have liked to have had as a parent. Some people, who are parents themselves, visualize their adult selves taking care of their child selves, saying, "I wish I'd had a parent like I am."

▶ **When I do the visualization and let myself experience the child, I get angry—very, very angry. How do I handle that?**

If you feel your anger could get out of control, protect yourself and others by doing the visualization with someone else present. A counselor can help you with this.

Often, however, we feel that any anger at all is a lot. This happens if we were raised with a prohibition on anger, or if we viewed a family member getting out of control with his anger. In that case, you might try feeling a little bit of it by yourself. But be kind to yourself, and call on a friend if you're concerned.

There is nothing wrong with screaming, shouting, or stomping your anger out. It's only a feeling. It's only anger. Try kicking a stone down the street, play racquetball or hand ball, throw a pillow, or say some four letter words.

► **Do I need to confront the people in real life who hurt me?**

No. Usually the hurt was done because of ignorance. You will be farther ahead in your healing process if you acknowledge the hurts and errors and absorb yourself in fixing them.

If your parents or teachers are open to learning, share the new information you have with them. Do this in a matter-of-fact way.

If you feel this sharing is not enough to satisfy you, then tell them how angry or hurt you were. Ask them if they realized how you felt. If they react poorly, continuing to blame or abuse you, then you may want to stand up for your inner child. Generally, however, angry confrontation is not at all necessary.

Remember, your main job is to heal yourself and take over responsibility for your growth.

► **Why is it so hard to forgive and go on?**

All of us have a hard time living with unfinished emotional business. Our emotions keep pulling us back to the problem in an attempt to get us to solve it. Usually we don't let go of a problem because there is some aspect that is not yet solved. People with ADD have to work hard to get past the point of hurt or blame and turn that energy into constructive action. But it's worth the effort.

► **How long will it take for my inner child to forgive those who abused me?**

It will take your child part as long as it needs to take. There is no point in pushing yourself. Do not let others try to tell you that you should forgive your abusers. It will simply happen when all the healing is done.

► **What if I can't get my child to forgive them?**

Often unexpressed anger stands in the way of being able to forgive someone. This is most likely to happen when we understand what happened to us but have not yet fully felt or acknowledged all the feelings within us. It's a matter of getting what we know cognitively to the level of feelings. Once the feelings are fully acknowledged and felt, and appropriate action is taken on behalf of them, the forgiveness will come.

► **How long will it take me to go through the grief process?**

Grieving also takes as long as it takes. A major grief reaction (to a divorce or death of a loved one) takes at least two years.

Recovery from the grief over your lost potential may go more quickly, provided you work with it. Doing the visualization work will facilitate your recovery, and it may only take a session or two to get beyond the feelings you've carried all these years.

► **What does it mean if I don't or can't feel any grief over my lost potential?**

You may have already gone through your grief. You certainly don't want to make up feelings you don't have.

► **How can I learn to let myself feel?**

Begin with another person who will help you realize when you are feeling. That person can be a counselor but doesn't necessarily have to be. She can be a friend who will stop you when you get an expression on your face or act in a way that tells her you are having strong feelings. You can then learn to identify what you are feeling.

► **If I start letting myself feel, will I still be able to work and stay in control of my life?**

Of course. In fact, you will be in even more control because it is an illusion that your feelings will go away if you don't acknowledge them. They actually only get more out of your control, doing their work behind the scenes.

To protect other areas of your life from the effects of your feelings, you can assign specific times to pay attention to them and to pay attention to work. Let your inner child know you will come back to the feelings at that specific time.

► **I'm shy in groups and wouldn't want to let other people know what I really feel. Can I fix myself in private?**

You can begin to work with your feelings in private, but ultimately you will need to openly acknowledge them. Being reticent to share feelings openly is one of the symptoms of the hurt and emotional damage you have suffered. Shame is one of the most common reactions to such hurt, leaving us feeling as if others would reject us or not want to be around us if they really knew what we felt or were like. Not so!

► **I get disgusted with myself for being so disorganized.**

What can I do to help myself?

First of all, quit being so abusive with yourself. You learned that as a child, and it's time to unlearn it. Realize that you do have innate forms of organization, but no one knows how to help you find them. All this time you've tried to learn ways that never fit you.

If all else fails, hire someone to keep track of your stuff or make a trade with someone who needs a skill you have.

▶ **If I don't feel comfortable doing the visualization, how can I feel better about myself?**

There are many ways to heal the past so you can move on to the future. You may be able to write out your healing. Try writing a letter to the child within you who suffered the repercussions of ADD. Also write letters to those who hurt you and to those who helped you. You can get your anger out this way and can even write a letter forgiving everyone involved, but only when you are good and ready.

I've known people who painted out their healing and others who used athletics, music, and drama. Anything goes. Use the mode that you feel drawn to.

▶ **Will the visualization conflict with what my counselor is having me do?**

I can't imagine how it would, regardless of the type of counseling you are undergoing. However, check with that person. He or she may even be able to help you visualize better.

▶ **How can I like the child part of me? She's so dumb.**

You have a good case of self-abuse going. Realize you

learned to feel that way and so you can unlearn it. Try getting a picture of yourself when you were about five or six. That's probably when you started school and began to have trouble with your ADD. Talk with the child in the picture.

Share the picture with someone you trust. Often a therapist can help you with this phase, especially if you have a tough case of "dumb feeling." As the other person loves your child, you will have a model to watch and imitate. The day will come, mark my words, when you will appreciate your child and understand the pain she's been through. You will then look at her as a courageous person who survived.

▶ **I can't get over feeling bad about having trouble in school and everyone blaming me.**

The most common block in this kind of situation is unexpressed anger. In your mind, call forth the people who offended you, and let the school child tell them off royally. Then, visualize the child going through school successfully, with understanding from the adults and other children. In fact, have them congratulate you on your assets while helping you cope with your ADD.

That ought to do the trick.

◄ı◄ı◄ 9 ı►ı►ı►

Restructuring

▼

Learning to successfully live with your ADD means not only repairing the emotional damage it has caused you, but also learning to manage your behavior to reflect your new self-image and to accomplish your new goals. Generally this means unlearning some old, bad habits and structuring your life and thinking to promote new ones. Controlling your temper, managing your time, and completing assigned tasks are top priorities. Here are ways to help you achieve follow-through, stick to an activity, handle distractions, reach the goals you set, and generally meet your special needs in both your personal world and the workplace.

► Cutting a Deal

Follow-through has been tough for you, since distractions pull you off course. In relationships, lack of follow-through destroys trust. Rarely have you meant to hurt others, but that is the effect nonetheless.

You'll find it helpful to cut a deal with anyone you're involved with, especially on a personal level, since you are likely to let down in the comfort of your personal life. Ask for reminders saying you really intend to follow through but tend to get off track, over-schedule, and under-organize. Also, take extra responsibility to remind yourself. You may add personal items

85

to your appointment book, mount a sign on your refrigerator, or do whatever works for you. Lists and schedules can be your best friends.

It's important to agree only to what you want to do. With your sensitivity, it's difficult for you to fake it effectively. You need to be honest.

▶ Pacing

It's a good idea for you to break each job into small, manageable segments that fit your attention span. For example, the yard may need to be mowed in three stages. In stage one, pick up all the things laying about, and then take a break to do whatever else you want for a short time. Then, in stage two, ready the lawn mower, which may include getting the gas for it. Give yourself a break to something not connected to the lawn, such as watching a TV show that has a clear ending time. This will be the time to return to work on the lawn. In stage three, mow the lawn. If it's a large lawn, mow it in sections according to a pre-arranged plan, taking a break between each section.

By structuring your breaks to fit your own timing, you are killing two birds with one stone: you're respecting your natural ability and you are putting yourself in charge of meeting your needs. Be sure you limit your breaks. You may want to get a timer. Or limit yourself to watching one half-hour TV show, or listening to one segment of a radio talk show, or reading one article in the newspaper. You may want to limit yourself to performing a single chore on the break—putting in the laundry or making a casserole for dinner.

No matter what the task, pacing is crucial for you. There is absolutely no point in pressing yourself to stick to a task. It's a better idea—and one that carries better odds for completion—to take a break when needed and as often as needed, and then go back to the task at hand. When control is in your hands, over time there will be an increase in attention to the task.

▶ Work Space

Develop a good relationship with your work area. Being pinned down in a small space with no ability to move about is a problem for most people with ADD. On the other hand, your need for structure and limits remains important. So, to accommodate both needs, I suggest a moderate size work space that allows opportunities to move in and out easily. It should be separated from the surrounding environment so that it blocks out noise and keeps visual distractions to a minimum. Cubicles work well for some people. Separate rooms are good for others. The worst environment for you, in all likelihood, is a large, noisy room with no barriers to screen out the environment.

▶ Movement

It's helpful for you to be able to move from one area of work to another during your time-out periods. It will help with the fidgets that likely affect you after you sit too long. This is one reason for taking breaks. If you're trapped in a lecture hall, take an end seat so you can get up and get a drink of water. It's also a good idea to have something to keep your hands busy.

▶ Sound

Sound screens are important. That's why having the TV or radio on in the background may be advantageous. At first it may seem like a distraction, but in reality, if the TV or music forms a kind of "white noise" with an even level of intensity, it actually covers up discrepant noises that can be a distraction. The hum of a ceiling fan or motor can do wonders to soothe and focus you.

Bottom line to your work environment: Allow yourself the freedom to work in the environment that feels best to you. Forget the guidelines generally taught in school or by parents. Your intuition knows better.

► Planning

You probably feel better, more secure, and capable of accomplishment by having a set pattern, at least for certain tasks. When I think of the way my son has learned to plan tasks, I'm always reminded of the pre-flight check that pilots go through before taking an airplane off the ground. They never deviate from the specific checklist and automatically adhere to it to provide safety for their passengers and themselves. Such patterned behavior may suit you very well. I strongly recommend integrating such patterns into every ordinary task, whether it's closing up the house at night or bathing the baby. It's important that you make up your own sequences, though, so they fit you.

► Mastering Distractions

Procrastination traditionally has been considered a fear or rebellion response: fear of failure or rebellion against a teacher, parent, or someone who pressed us to do something we didn't want to do.

But we're not dealing with tradition here. We're dealing with ADD. Yes, while you may be more susceptible to the fear of failure because you've had more experience with it, and you may have found yourself a rebel, there's an additional reason why you may *appear* to procrastinate: distractibility.

You can change that, for delivering the goods on time is part of your new self-image, isn't it?

It's crucial for you to have an outline for any project and—preferably—an appointment book or daily schedule with the patterns for work clearly laid out.

Despite a lot of talk to the contrary, ADD people are really no different from anyone else when it comes to avoiding work they don't want to do but feel they should. You may be hit harder by it than your fellow heel-diggers, though, because it's characteristically much more difficult for you to concentrate on something you don't want to do (remember, this is one of the diagnostic criteria). But, to live in this world, you must commit to doing some of these "should" tasks. Make them part of your own agenda.

If the checkbook needs to be balanced, it's important to know what the advantages are for doing the balancing. Then check for an inner willingness to take on the job as something that is in your best interest—not because someone says it ought to be done. If you can't find a reason, then don't do it: hire someone to do it, or trade with your partner or spouse for another task.

Leave more time to get distracted—often. That's one way. But I also recommend leaving a shorter time to finish a project, carefully and thoroughly structuring the time, and then going for broke. In other words, let yourself procrastinate. The condensed time frame will make you focus more intensely on the project, and all extraneous activities can be let go—whew! No dishes or yard work allowed.

It works. One of my patients and I structured her school semester as the chart on the next page shows. Just as I helped her, you may wish to have a buddy help you. The chart came about with four weeks left in the term. Five papers were due, six exams were coming up, and she still had to attend classes. As you can see, even though we eliminated all unnecessary activities, we still scheduled some TV time. The reward was 17 credits of straight A's for my client. I rest my case! I have included other sample charts as well.

▶ Getting Your Temper under Control

The earlier temper control is begun, the easier it is to effect alternative ways for its management. A temper is something that lives only through reinforcement. It can be controlled in the child if the child is taught to find other means to get his or her needs met. But, because that rarely happens, let's pick up on the adult level, learning how to break the temper cycle.

DAILY ACTIVITY SCHEDULE

NAME: Jane Sample   DATE:

DESCRIPTION: full time student (straight A record) who works 8hrs per week

	MONDAY	TUESDAY	WEDNESDAY	THURSDAY	FRIDAY	SATURDAY	SUNDAY
7:00 am	Pack Lunch Eat, Watch TV	Pack Lunch, Eat	Pack Lunch Eat, Watch TV	Pack Lunch Eat	Pack Lunch Eat, watch TV	TV or sleep in work	Eat Lightly Read Book
8:00 am	Drive time	Drive to school Study at	Drive time	Drive to school Study at	Drive Time		Alcoholics Anonymous
9:00 am	Physical Education	school	Physical Education	school	Physical Education		
10:00 am	Change Clothes 10:15 School Counselor	Lab 10:30-History	Change Clothes Errands	LAB 10:30-History	Change Clothes Errands		10:30-Lunch
11:00 am	Lab		Lab		Lab	Shopping and Chores	
12:00 noon	Logic	Sociology	Logic	Sociology	Logic		Study or Library
1:00 pm	1:30-Spanish	1:30-English	1:30 Spanish	1:30 English	1:30-spanish	Library and Computer time with breaks	and Computer Time with
2:00 pm			Drive Time		Free	as long as needed	breaks
3:00 pm	3:30-Snack	Study	3:30-Counsellor	Library	Time		
4:00 pm	Study		Drive Time 4:30-Free time	Drive Time work			
5:00 pm				Drive time			Dinner with a friend
6:00 pm	Dinner Drive	Dinner and Drive time	Dinner	Dinner		Dinner with friends	6:30 Plan next week
7:00 pm	Study with walking breaks		Study	Study		a movie or hang out	Finish study projects
8:00 pm		Alcoholics Anonymous					
9:00 pm	Watch TV	Drive time					
10:00 pm	Bed and Relaxation Time	Bed and relaxation time	10:30-Bed and relaxation time	10:30 Bed and relaxation time	Bed and relaxation time	10:30 Bed and relaxation time	Bed and relaxation time
11:00 pm							
12:00 midnight							

5/7 - 5/11

5/14 - 5/21

Mon
10:30 And.
1p Station
6:30 Aerobics

Books
2 Good 4 Dm Good
Slept D
Water Up Sleep Beach
32 Elephant Peanuts

Tues 9a Hair
1p WSRT 600-0000
Call Bob @ Network
6:30p Aerobics

Wed
12a meeting w/ producer
1p Station
Send card to boss (ratings)

Thurs. 7:30-8 Firestone
8:45 Breakfast
12a P/u car
1p Station

Fri 11:30 Mike J.
1p Station
6:30 Aerobics

Sat 1p John - Hair
Call producer

Mon
1p Station
5p Lee Burnett - Balcom

Tues
8:30 And.
Call John A@ 611-1111
1p Station

Wed
1p Station

Thurs
1p Station

Fri
1p Station

MONTHLY PLANNER Preferred by a 35 year old male salesman.

MONTH ___Sept.___

MONDAY	TUESDAY	WEDNESDAY	THURSDAY	FRIDAY	SATURDAY	SUNDAY
	☺ Dancing	Pay bills		☺ Lunch with mother		yard
	☺ Dancing		Community meeting		~~Work~~	~~Work~~
WORK project due	☺ DANCING	Pay bills		prepare work for trip		PACK Leave
Out of town ————→			————→	John's 10th b-day party ☺		yard
write	☺ DANCING	write	write	Turn in written proposal	Dinner/Theatre boss	

DAILY ACTIVITY SCHEDULE

NAME:_____   DATE:_____

DESCRIPTION:_____

	MONDAY	TUESDAY	WEDNESDAY	THURSDAY	FRIDAY	SATURDAY	SUNDAY
7:00 am							
8:00 am							
9:00 am							
10:00 am							
11:00 am							
12:00 noon							
1:00 pm							
2:00 pm							
3:00 pm							
4:00 pm							
5:00 pm							
6:00 pm							
7:00 pm							
8:00 pm							
9:00 pm							
10:00 pm							
11:00 pm							
12:00 midnight							

Remember, that temper gets a particular hold on ADD people because of the tendency for emotional flooding to occur. So, step one is: never try to deal with a temper when it is active. Make plans when all is calm, cool, and collected. Acknowledge that you have a temper. Forget the business of blaming others. To be sure, someone cutting in front of you on the freeway may have triggered your anxiety, surprised you, or frightened you, but your particular reaction of temper is *your* responsibility. You must realize that there are other ways to react to the stress. And with your willingness, you can learn alternatives that work particularly well for you in dealing with family and work settings, the places where temper is most likely to work against you.

1) Decide on a signal that means it's time to stop whatever is going on. In our house, it's the "time-out" sign used in sports. Anyone in the family can use it and we automatically stop—no questions asked. The questions can come later. This time-out breaks into the flooding and stops the emotions from taking over. Practically, this type of thing will work in a family setting, but what about when someone pulls in front of you in traffic? What do you do then? Pull your car over to the side of the road if necessary. If you're at the office, take a walk if you can, or go to the restroom and wash your face. Go outside. The point is, *stop the emotional flooding.* If others are around, tell them you'll be back in a little while. Go to the store for milk if you have to. If it is your partner who's having the trouble, be nonchalant with other people and just say, "He's taking a break." No one will notice if the emotional level is held down.

2) Identify the feeling underlying the anger—fear, frustration, helplessness, hopeless—and use words to express that feeling.

"I feel helpless in this situation."

"I felt frightened when that car pulled out in front of me."

"I feel put down by you."

Be honest. It may be hard at first, but is pays off once you've learned to do it. Start by making the statements to yourself, if it's too difficult to do so with others initially.

3) Ask yourself two simple questions: "What do I need to feel better or become a winner here? How can I get it?"

4) Give yourself permission to get whatever it is you want (certainly within socially acceptable limits). Power in a situation is a common need, and you must take it to get your needs met.

5) Promise yourself that you will continue to work to get what you want without throwing a temper tantrum.

6) Congratulate yourself on a job well done.

You'll be surprised how quickly you can break the temper cycle by following these steps. It is not a long, trying process—unless someone around you enables you to continue with your temper or even cultivates it by reinforcing it. They do you no favor but probably don't know any better, so you might as well make up your mind to open up alternatives in spite of them.

Every time someone gives in to your temper, you end up a loser. Every time someone scolds you or gives any attention to your temper, you end up a loser. You're no loser, so stop giving your power away to others. Get it through your head that you're a winner and deserve to be one.

What do you do, though, if you are waiting on a customer and he becomes angry and unfairly challenges you? The first reaction of a person with ADD would be to fight back. But that's definitely nonconstructive for business. So you need a quick fix technique—a way to deflect your anger immediately and keep it from escalating until you have the time to sort yourself out and follow the steps above. Try a stop-review-go approach to such situations:

Put a "stop" sign where you can see it—a sticker on the cash register, say, or a little trinket on your watchband. When something happens, glance at it and visualize yourself stopping your temper, as you would a car at an intersection. Use the sports time-out sign if you want.

Quickly, during this mental pause, look over a couple of acceptable options to blowing your top or striking out. It could be just a smile and an offer to get the manager, or an offer to help the customer put the complaint in writing. Once you've begun collecting options to temper as you retrain yourself, they will come rather quickly.

Now, go ahead and release yourself to exercise the option you chose.

▶ Common Questions about Restructuring

> ▶ **How do I quit taking the lack of follow-through by my friend with ADD personally? It makes me feel as if the person doesn't really care about me.**
>
> Your reaction is very normal. To overcome it, use your brain to begin to change how you feel. Realize mentally that the lack of follow-through is often an attribute of ADD. Talk to yourself, saying, "It's not me that's causing the problem. My friend does care about me." It will take a little time, but I would expect your feelings to listen. If they don't, then you probably felt uncared for as a child, and this behavior by your friend is triggering old

memories that you need to work with.

► **If I agree to only what I want to do, my wife calls me selfish. And I feel selfish. Isn't it wrong to be selfish?**

Selfishly eating the last piece of cake without sharing it with others in the room is quite different from taking care of yourself. I'm talking about taking responsibility for getting your own needs met. If you will do that, then you will be in a much better place to take care of others who truly cannot take care of themselves, such as people who are sick, or children.

To consistently do for another person what they can do for themselves cheats them of the wonderful reward of being responsible. You wouldn't want to do that, would you?

► **It makes me mad to have trouble keeping my attention on a job. What can I do about my bad feelings?**

First check to see whether you are trying to do a job that doesn't fit you.

Acknowledge to yourself that it is a nuisance having to accommodate your ADD in such situations. Get those feelings out. Then, congratulate yourself for doing the job anyway.

Say, "There goes that ADD of mine again." Then laugh and say, "And I'm learning to work with it even in situations that don't fit. Good for me."

► **Isn't being controlling a bad way to be?**

Being controlling has earned a bad name these days. A controlling person tries to control what other people do as well as the outcomes of anything he or she is involved with. That's not the same as being *in control.*

To be *in control* means we are able to take responsibility for ourselves and our behavior, neither blaming others nor circumstances for our difficulties or inadequacies. We also know when we are incapable of accomplishing whatever we desire and we purposely let go of control, at least for a period of time. There is a conscious, thought-through decision, taking into account all information at our disposal, before we decide to change our pathway or even quit.

There is nothing bad about being *in control.*

► **If I have to sit and listen during meetings at work, it makes me feel awful trying to stay still. I feel like I want to jump out of my skin but I need to look professional. What can I tell my boss or colleague if I take in something to keep my hands busy?**

Simply say you concentrate better when your hands are occupied and leave it at that.

► **Why does playing with a paper clip or hand-held water toy help me stay still?**

It gives you something to focus your attention on almost hypnotically. By doing this, you are less likely to be distracted by other things that are going on around you. It is soothing to the nerves and allows you to focus on the main agenda.

► **Which kind of chart should I use to keep track of my time?**

Different people with ADD respond to different types of charts. You will need to experiment. If you use one that is highly structured, it is important that you be the one to decide what goes into it rather than have someone else tell you what should be there. Some people do better starting each day with a blank page and making a list of what is to be done.

► **My spouse has an awful temper but blames me for causing it. What can I do to avoid triggering it? Is there anything I can do to take the steam out of his temper if he won't work on it?**

When you two are in a clam mood, ask him what hurt him. Then, practice saying things in a matter-of-fact way. Know, however, that he needs to take responsibility for his display of temper.

Do not reinforce his temper. When he blasts off, do not argue. The most you want to say is, "I'll talk with you when you're calm." You may need to wait until he is calm to say this.

Most people with tempers will display just as much temper as they can get away with. So, if you don't like the temper outbursts, tell him you are simply unwilling to put up with them. Tell him what will happen when he allows his temper to get out of control. You might way, "When you yell, I'm going to leave the house. I'll return when you speak in a normal voice." Then, you must be willing to follow through. You will find that you can set the limit anywhere you want and, if you mean it, the person will adjust his behavior.

► **I used to have a temper but it is much better now that I've been working on it. My husband still reacts as if I have one though, tiptoeing around on eggshells. How can I get him to stop?**

Ask him, "What will it take to get you to relax? I've changed and I need you to catch up with my changes." Do realize, though, that it may take several months for him to catch up. It won't happen all in one day, either.

So some patience on your part is wise. On the other hand, if your husband continues to walk on eggshells, you may need to set a limit on his behavior by saying, "Hey, cut it out. I'm getting turned off. I'm even beginning to wonder whether you want my temper back."

► **Are there certain circumstances when an ADD person's temper will be more likely to erupt even after control measures have been learned?**

Tiredness is the biggest culprit I know. Also, keep track of the amount of stress that you are under. Times of change are high stress times and likely circumstances for an explosion.

Occasionally a resistant temper indicates an organic problem, such as a seizure disorder. Referral for a neuropsychological workup is in order.

◄ı◄ı◄10ı►ı►ı►

For Family and Friends

▼

M y heart goes out to parents who are frustrated beyond words, trying to *get* their offspring to act responsibly.

We all lose it at times, berating our sons and daughters out of our own sense of helplessness, but for parents of an ADD child or young adult, the trials are particularly painful and frustrating. Believe me, I know.

ADD may keep parents from having the kind of child they expected and wanted. We parents are under terrific peer pressure to have our children, as an extension of ourselves, perform up to cultural standards, and we often pass the pressure on to our kids. We expect them to produce so we can feel acceptable. We make them responsible for our achievements as parents.

As if that's not enough, we expect them to achieve by being taught in a particular way. Heaven help the child with ADD who cannot readily screen out external stimuli. He is still placed in a classroom with twenty-five or more other kids and told it's his responsibility to pay attention.

Ideally, we won't permit such abuse—and we won't commit it, either. If we had known of the ADD, we would have evaluated the child in light of all his skills and limitations and then provided an environment supportive of the child's needs so blossoming could occur. Our job—to ignore peer pressure and prepare an environment that is supportive of growth—would have been carried out with care and love. Most of us never did this.

Leave your guilt behind. You did the best you could. But realize any adult child will need help to overcome the repercussions of the abuse. Even lack of understanding is perceived as abuse, as I'm using the term.

It's crucial to realize that a person is not bad because he has a temper outburst, is unable to stick to a task, or impulsively changes plans. It's a nuisance to live with these behaviors, but we must distinguish between the person and the behavior. None of us is so perfect that we can stand in judgment of others. What we can do is say "no" to behaviors. We can even reject behaviors while understanding the source of them.

A simple response like, "I understand you're angry, but, no, you may not hit me," seems like no more than common sense, but in fact reflects a good deal of self-control and understanding.

▶ Parenting Your ADD Child

The trick to completing the childrearing process of an ADD young adult is fairly simple, if a few rules are followed:

1) Intervene with the outside world on behalf of the ADD child as much as is needed when the child is young, and then slow down each year.

2) Similarly, give your ADD child increasing responsibility with each year and let him know you believe he can handle it.

3) Let go of your dreams for your son's or daughter's potential. Instead, seek to uncover his or her dreams. Then support them. Just because your ADD child shows

102

natural ability with numbers doesn't mean he can or would want to become an accountant. Quit pushing and let him use his number skills to become a topnotch salesperson, or whatever he wants to become.

4) Let your ADD young adult follow a creative path toward adulthood. Just because everyone else in the family has a college degree doesn't mean your grown child has to have one too. Let go, I'm not saying persons with ADD can't make it in college but only that the decision needs to fit the person.

5) Give your child your belief in his ability to do well by and for himself. Not only is such belief a precious gift, it also sets up a greater likelihood of success.

6) If your adult ADD child is acting irresponsibly or destructively, let him be responsible for the consequences of his action. You don't need to get into punishing him for misdeeds or irresponsibility. Rather, simply allow natural consequences to fall where they may. Do not bail your son or daughter out of trouble. Stand by his side, however, while he bails himself out of trouble. For example, don't have your attorney get your child out of a DWI charge. Instead, offer to help him get help. Go to court with him, or be available to talk and plan if your child wishes. Go to Al-Anon and give him the AA number. But don't be a pest on any of the issues. Make the offer; then back off.

Parenting the adult ADD child is simple in concept but tough in execution because you must overcome your own weaknesses and vulnerabilities. You have to learn to say "no" and be willing to let go of control. He may do things differently than you would have, but who says your way is right for everyone?

If you are having difficulty being firm, you may want to ask a friend to give you some help. If you start to weaken, say, in response to a request for money, call your friend and say, "I'm thinking of giving him more money." Your friend can take you out to lunch until the urge passes.

▶ Parents, Siblings, and ADD

Realistically, brothers and sisters will fuss and fight to some degree. But ADD often multiplies the conflicts, sometimes unbearably, and complicates the sibling relationships to the extent that special effort must be made to keep balance and harmony amongst brothers and sisters. A few simple—and not so simple—strategies for parents to follow when children are young:

1) Basically ignore their antics unless one sibling consistently takes advantage of the other. There is a good deal more sibling abuse—verbal, sexual, and physical—than meets the eye, and it occurs when one sibling characteristically takes advantage of the other. How do you tell what's really going on? You may need to play detective to decide. Do a bit of eavesdropping, like a fly on the wall. Listen to both sides of the story, and be careful that the more articulate, calmer person isn't the one believed all the time.

2) Set up situations where cooperation reaps more rewards than conflict does. For example, walk away from them when they begin to argue; pay attention and praise them when they cooperate.

3) Expect one sibling to behave better than the other for periods of time and then expect roles to be reversed. This is just a normal part of daily living. Even though one may have ADD and will often have special needs, the other—the so-called "normal" one—will also have good days and bad days. Just because one child has ADD doesn't mean the other is a saint.

4) Teach each child to use words to tell you what he wants. Help the ADD child who is impulsive learn to take time to get the words out and take time to get his needs met. And how do you do that? By showing him that words work. Be very patient. Wait for the child to speak his

104

piece; take time to understand what he's trying to say.

5) Teach the children how each person is different—not better or worse. And teach them how they can use their differences to help one another if they cooperate. Teach them what ADD is and how it works.

6) Reinforce how families stick together to help one another, and how brothers and sisters can fuss sometimes but still respect each other's differences.

▶ Adult Siblings and ADD

Now let's suppose this groundwork had not been laid. It's never too late to learn. As they get older, one sibling can approach the other and begin to get acquainted.

The one with ADD may want to share the new information being learned, for once ADD is identified, they can both talk about its effects rather than the person.

At times it's a nuisance to be ADD, and it's a nuisance to live with a person with Attention Deficit Disorder. Siblings shared hard times from different sides of the table. Each sibling may want to share feelings, even grieve together a little, for both lost something in their relationship. Each can share what he or she likes about the other's skills, what's admired and respected. They might agree on a cue, like the time-out signal, to be used when either sibling is getting frustrated. (We're assuming here that all parties have been informed of the ADD and believe in it, which, of course, is part of your job as a successful family leader.)

Don't get me wrong. ADD will still be a factor. Personality differences may still make it difficult for siblings to work together. But reconciling over the ADD does bring understanding and empathy,. and don't underestimate the power of understanding: It supports love.

▶ Try Negotiating

Blaming can be such a large part of an ADD person's life—and the lives of those who live with him—that learning negotiating skills is not only desirable but necessary.

Whether you are a friend, parent, spouse, or ADD person, follow these guidelines:

- ▶ Remember that it doesn't matter why something happened.

- ▶ But it does matter what happened.

- ▶ Therefore, eliminate all judgment from your discussions. (Later, you can work on eliminating judgment from your thoughts, too.)

- ▶ Get to the facts.

- ▶ Come up with a plan to solve the problem rather than worry how the problem got there. Be specific in your plan.

- ▶ Lay out specific ways to accomplish the steps in your plan.

- ▶ Set the plan in motion, one step at a time, and stick to it at all costs. You'll get used to negotiating your needs, and you will end up feeling like, and being, a winner in the long run.

As explained in the previous chapter, follow-through can be tough for someone with ADD, since distractions have the effect of pulling us off course. In relationships, lack of follow-through destroys trust. Rarely does an ADD person mean to hurt you, but that is the effect nonetheless. The point is: Don't take lack of follow-through personally. It's only a symptom of ADD, not lack of caring or love.

Whether you are the ADD person or the person who lives with him, it is helpful to negotiate a deal, since the comfort of closeness in a relationship is likely to lead to a let-down in diligence. We all often behave the worst around those we love the most.

Ask for permission to issue reminders. (Don't just assume them as your right.) The person reminding should recognize that the ADD person sincerely intends to follow through but should also recognize the tendency to get off-track. Both you and the ADD person have to take extra responsibility in this. Bearing in mind that lists and schedules can be the ADD person's best friends, you might help in posting them, making sure they're up to date, and, with the agreement of the ADD person, seeing that they're adhered to. (It's best if the ADD person himself makes the lists. Personal experience has taught me that this is the most effective way for lists to work.)

Be sure, if you are the spouse, friend, or parent of an ADD person, that you depersonalize the experience and that you omit anger from your interaction. A tall order? You bet, and one that takes practice to deliver. But you can do it, once your expectations come in line with the reality of ADD. It won't be immediate, but once you've relinquished your need to have your expectations met (and who said they weren't loaded with your own dysfunctions?), you can reassure the ADD person that it's okay to say "no" if the person doesn't want to do whatever you ask. The next time your ADD person says "no" to your request, say a big "thank you" for his being honest.

When there is a lack of follow-through in a particular situation, nicely and gently be sure that "yes" was intended when the commitment was made. If "yes" remains the answer, then ask "when" again in an anger-free tone. Or maybe ask "how" the person intends to follow through. Set a time line acceptable to both of you. If the time elapses without the ADD person completing the task, do it yourself—be it finding a companion for a movie or mowing the lawn—rather than becoming bitter or resentful.

Continuing to try to get someone to follow through only leads to frustration and, frankly, it's important once the negotiation stage has passed to simply remember to stop expecting follow-through. Don't start from this point, but do end at this point if practice doesn't lead to success.

For the ADD person, there are ramifications and responsibilities to the negotiation process. After reassurances that only commitments will be made where the follow-through is intended, it's very important that the ADD person indeed follow through. The willingness to try must be negotiated once and for all. Individual situations must be negotiated as needed. There are times, even when you try your best with an ADD person, when they fail, to follow through. And if they fail, don't blame yourself for permanent damage to trust in the relationship. Of course, it may not mean loss of the relationship entirely, but no one will blame you for seeing him—or her—as someone who cannot be trusted to live up to commitments.

Grief on your part over that loss is common and, in fact, some of the anger that occurs is a part of the grief reaction.

▶ Dealing with Rigidity

The sensitivity of ADD people makes them prone to put down or overreact in pressure or surprise situations. And the surprises don't have to be unpleasant ones. I remember well one birthday when I thought it would be fun to put special candles on the cake of an ADD person—candles that couldn't be blown out. I didn't know at the time that the person had ADD and, anyway, wouldn't have expected the result I got, which was anger, at the surprise and at me. I didn't understand at the time why my attempt to bring fun to the party backfired. Now I understand.

To say with a sharp agitated voice, "Quick, we're late. I just looked at my watch and we're already late," is to court resistance and irritation. The ADD person is likely to look at you with disdain or even anger. The more you prod, force, or become hysterical, the more he will resist.

So, difficult as it may be, force yourself to be calm. Explain the situation. In fact, asking the ADD person calmly for help is much more likely to yield a positive response. It may take a few more minutes in the beginning—and tons more effort on your part—but the results in the long term will more than offset your initial frustration. Don't worry if you slip up sometimes. I know how it feels because I get scared and frantic sometimes, and in so doing become my own worst enemy. Forget your errors, for they are part and parcel of living, and strive simply to do the best you can. It's a tall order, but you can do it.

► Living

Living with someone who has ADD takes lots of understanding on both sides, much ability to trust in one another's best intentions, and lots of negotiation skills. As long as each person is good of heart, and willing to take responsibility, letting the other work on himself, the relationship has a good prognosis. If one person needs to be over-controlling or particularly needs to keep the ADD person inadequate, then a healthy relationship is a lot less likely. The merits of the relationship need to be reconsidered under these circumstances.

Quality relationships can survive—and flourish—when there are two winners and no losers. This takes seeing the other's point of view, communicating on understanding of that viewpoint, and seeking a resolution without stopping until you find a mutually suitable solution that you both can live with. Good luck, and keep at it until you find the answer.

► Common Questions from Friends and Family Members

> ► I feel very guilty about what we did and allowed to be done to our son when he was a child. Is there anything we can do to feel better? And what can we do for our son?

109

For yourself, please be forgiving. Know that you did the very best you could do at the moment you were doing it. Had you known a better way, you'd have used it.

For your son, sit down with him and tell him of your new awareness. Give him information. Tell him you think he did a tremendous job surviving thus far and that you would like to support him. And you might want to help him get some relearning if he would like to. There's nothing wrong with including financial support for schooling or retraining, if he requests it or accepts your offer accompanied with a plan and follow-through.

Don't overdo to make up for the past. Don't take responsibility to fix him now because you feel guilty. Rather, form a partnership with him in which he does all he can do and you help out where you can. You may want a counselor to help you determine where the line between helping and enabling lies.

▶ **Why does my ADD husband get all his jobs done at work and fails to get anything finished at home? He's either a couch potato watching TV or he's asleep.**

It is not unusual for adults with ADD to use up all their energy focusing their attention at work. By the time they get home, there's no energy left for goal directed behavior.

Don't take his behavior personally or think he doesn't care. Talk with him about setting aside a specific time, after a rest, to do one thing at a time. Let him know it would really help you.

It also might be a great help to do some chores together. Team work often is effective in helping the ADD person stay centered on an activity.

▶ **Why do I have to renegotiate every little situation with my spouse? Is she just pretending to agree with me to get me off her back?**

In all likelihood not. It's important to determine whether your wife intends to cooperate with you and simply forgets or gets distracted or whether she is indeed just agreeing to get you off her back.

You must make it safe for her to be honest with you, which includes saying "no." Tell her that and make sure the next "no" is greeted with, "I'm glad you're telling me when you don't want to do something."

▶ **From the sound of things, my non-diagnosed adult ADD son married a non-diagnosed adult ADD woman. I've never understood how they can have such verbal uproars and then make up in a little while. What can they do?**

Very possibly their uproars bother you more than them. Theirs is a common pattern when two people with ADD find each other. It's wonderful or awful. But remember, they probably understand each other on a very deep level, because of their shared ADD. They would, though, both benefit from some training to find other ways to communicate that might be less emotionally charged. But that has to be left up to them.

▶ **What is the likelihood that they will have an ADD child?**

Fairly good. The research is not completely in yet, so I can't give you a definitive answer. They would, however, do well to acquire some skills before they bring a child into the situation, ADD or not.

▶ **Why is it better if the person with ADD makes up the reminder's list?**

Because a person with ADD feels everything acutely, he does better when he's in control of what affects him. Making up that list puts the power in the right hands.

▶ **How do I "depersonalize" my experience trying to negotiate with someone who's ADD?**

▶ Use your brain instead of your feelings.

▶ Think about what is happening.

▶ Think about what you would like to happen.

▶ Be aware of your expectations.

▶ Be aware of what you are feeling: fear, frustration, helplessness.

▶ Take responsibility for your feelings and learn what you need to do in order to attend to them.

▶ Enter your negotiations with a clear mind and settled feelings.

▶ **I'm sick and tired of making all the adjustments to my spouse's ADD. What options do I have?**

Sounds like you need to do some self-nurturing and spend extra time getting your needs met. You may have been depending on him or her too much and ended up out in the cold. Though you can understand your spouse's ADD, you do not have to acquire it.

Be a bit more selfish. For example: Let's say your family has decided to have a garage sale. You ended up with the job of labeling all the items even though you hate doing it. But you took the job because you were afraid it wouldn't get done if left to your distractible ADD spouse. You want to be able to talk to the people coming by, too, instead of doing the awful job. My advice to you is drop the labeling and go talk to people. Get a friend who owes you a favor to help with the labeling so it gets

112

done. Or label your own items and leave your spouse's unlabeled unless he does it. Keep the money from your things for yourself.

▶ **Even though I understand a lot more about ADD, my heart is burned out. Can I rekindle my love for my husband?**

Unfortunately that's a little hard to tell. In my years of counseling, I've seen fairly cool ashes rekindled. I've also seen people who chose to go their separate ways and were glad they did so.

You need to get rather philosophical about this. If it's meant to be, it will be. In the meantime, don't try to force anything. Pressure is the kiss of death. Look for little things to enjoy in each other and see what happens. Be open to feel the sweetness of love. It can happen.

▶ **My wife left me because of my irresponsibility. Now, I believe I am ADD. Our marriage never had a chance. How do I get over feeling awful about what happened?**

Attend to the grieving over the loss. Then find out all you can about ADD. Be properly diagnosed, join a support group, and start a new life for yourself. Learn, from this day forward, to make the most of what you have at any given moment. And learn from your experience so you don't make the same mistakes again.

▶ **If I don't take care of things around the house, the bills will never get paid, the repairs won't be made, and grass won't get mowed. I don't want to be codependent, but I'm tired of doing it all myself. Help!**

Do what you want to do for yourself and then give yourself a break. Reward yourself. Do not do for the person who is not holding up his or her share of the work load. If that person's unpicked-up clothing litters your living space and causes you to feel pain, ask him to pick it up and if he doesn't, either do it for yourself or pay to have it done and send him the bill. (Don't forget those to-do lists.)

Sadly, it is quite possible to love someone but not find them to be a compatible roommate. Set your priorities in order and make sure you get what you need most out of the relationship.

▶ **Why don't people with ADD like surprises?**

Surprises are intrusive. Sensitive people are going to feel the intrusion in extra measure. They also interrupt the steady flow of regularity. Remember people with ADD feel better and do better when they can count on what is going to happen.

▶ **If there's an emergency, what is the best way to get a person with ADD to react FAST?**

Act as calmly as you can. In a very matter-of-fact way, convey the information about the emergency directly to the person from close range in a moderate to low voice. Try not to hell across the room. Measure your words, telling the person what you need for him to do. Asking someone who's ADD to help you rather than giving direction is much more helpful in a crisis. Most people with ADD also like to know why they are being asked to do something. "I need you to immediately leave the house because it is on fire. If you will close the closet door, I will shut off the kitchen door and meet you outside."

◄ ◄ **11** ► ►

For Intimate Couples

▼

Achieving and maintaining an intimate relationship, both emotionally and physically, can be quite a challenge for both the ADD person and the significant other. But, with an understanding of the ground rules—what works and what doesn't—the return on the effort is highly rewarding.

► What Not To Do

It's very easy in an ADD relationship to form codependent behavior. Simply put, the individuals focus their attention on each other rather than taking responsibility for themselves. In this scenario, an ADD person is likely to blame everyone or everything around for his problems, and the ADD person's significant other is likely to take responsibility for all the problems and for the necessary corrections.

"If only I'd remembered to remind her to make the bank deposit, her checks wouldn't have bounced," might be a typical line. Any time you hear a question like, "What can *I* do to get *her* to be more responsible?" it's a sure sign of enabling behavior. And, the person with ADD may blame the other person, too, demanding, "Why didn't you remind me?"

In such an unhealthy relationship, the partner of an ADD person often carries the role of the "responsible" one, the fixer who parents everyone. Growing up he or she may have been the one who could quiet Daddy down when he drank too much. Or maybe that person held Mommy's hand during a thunderstorm when Mommy was thirty-seven and the child was three. Fixers need to be needed, usually are controlling, and run things in an organized manner. But things had better be done their way—or else. It takes a lot of courage to let an ADD person mind his own business while the fixer finds other ways to feel valuable and lovable.

Usually it's easier to fix and complain and baby the ADD person.

Such mutual dependency tends to keep couples stuck—and I mean stuck—together, each attracted to the other because of feelings of inadequacy. Usually, too, people stuck in such a relationship are disappointed in each other because someone else can't fix their lives for them.

▶ Good Things To Do

But there are ways to avoid codependency and still be supportive of your ADD partner and of yourself, behaviors that you can use immediately to see improvement.

It's difficult to overestimate the value of one technique: If you live with an ADD person, ask him or her questions. It helps the ADD person to process information. The questioning has to be done pointedly, but very gently, in a nonaccusatory way. The technique works especially well when the ADD partner is flooded, overwhelmed by the booming, buzzing world. "I've had it happen so many times when I'm flooded with information. I'm thinking of so many options that I can't do anything except yell or stomp off or shut down," says an ADD person. "When this happens, what usually works is for my mate to say 'What are you feeling right now? Tell me what you're thinking and we can go through the options one by one.' This kind of approach helps me focus on what I really want to do instead of being bombarded by a thousand other things."

There's something that the ADD partner can do to help take the frustration out of the relationship: Take the initiative in dealing constructively with the "hardness" of tasks. How do you tell your loved one when something is too hard for you because of your ADD? The best way is to be blunt and ask for understanding from your mate. "This is too hard for me because of my ADD," is a positive way to put it. It's not an admission of weakness, but, rather, of individual needs. And it could apply to no more than reading a map or picking from one of several spots to view wildflowers. At times when the ADD partner is overwhelmed, it's very helpful for the mate to say "Is there anything I can do to help you? What if we took it a piece at a time?" Or, "Do you just need to let the task go for now?"

Sound like codependency? Maybe, but it's not, and it's important for both of you to understand this. As the ADD person, you're asking for help, and in so doing, you're acting responsibly by looking after your needs, a very healthy action to take. As the partner of the person with ADD, you don't do any part of the task for the ADD adult that he can do for himself. Neither do you take responsibility without being asked or do anything you don't want to do.

The result of these efforts will be a new-found emotional intimacy where both partners feel safe, appreciated, and accepted. You'll be able to shift gears and share secrets and tell each other intimate and personal thoughts—and each of you will be able to ask for help without feeling vulnerable or codependent.

Married women with ADD are at a special disadvantage in this society. Traditionally, women handle a lot of the detail work in the running of a household—running the kids to and fro, planning the meals, coordinating timetables and the thousand little details that make up daily life—but this is precisely the area where ADD people need the most help. Imposing responsibility for these details, without help or the knowledge that ADD is present, can create a frustrating and hopeless situation for the woman in the family. What appears to be a simple and easily managed average day can be a nightmare for these women. If they can't ask their mate for help, who can they ask?

▶ Touching

We've talked before about touching and the special problems— and pleasures—it can present for a person with ADD. Frequently, someone who's ADD doesn't want to be touched at all; it causes pain. But, how do you tell someone close that you can't handle being touched right now, without hurting his or her feelings? When the partner needs or wants the contact, what can the person with ADD do that won't upset his partner but instead will convey a feeling of caring? One option to start with is the direct approach followed by saying what you can manage: "I'm feeling too sensitive right now. Could I just hold your hand or give you a quick hug, or just sit next to you?"

One woman wouldn't hug a man who had no awareness of his own strength. He'd always hurt her, even though she had told him many times that he was hurting her. His hugging felt painful to her. He just couldn't appreciate her sensitivity. So, she ducked his hugs and smiled a lot. Through small nuances and non-verbal communication, an ADD person often senses the ulterior motives of the person doing the hugging. The most common is a hidden sexual agenda. Generally, this kind of covert behavior breeds rejection, for she won't want to be touched by him.

Rhythmic touching, such as repetitive stroking or patting, usually annoys an ADD person. In its place, try gently and firmly taking an arm or a toe or one finger instead of a whole hand.

Although massages—the full-body type—may help reduce tension in many of us, they may be just too much of a good thing to some ADD people. The touch of the therapist is all important. If you and your ADD mate want to try massage as a pleasure-giving intimacy, try using oils to create a non-irritating touch, and keep the massage shorter, maybe to 30 minutes or so.

Experiment with variations. Once something pleasant is discovered, there is a strong possibility that the ADD person will not want to stick with it for very long. In turn, you may find it difficult to believe that the non-ADD partner likes the same thing repeatedly. Partners of ADD persons often find this phenomenon frustrating and have trouble getting the ADD person to repeat pleasurable touching.

Other Tips: Try hugging from behind instead of from the front. Or try putting the head of the ADD person in your lap. But be careful when you put your arm over the shoulder of an ADD person, especially a woman. The weight may feel too heavy.

▶ What About Sex?

Sex—so individual that it's difficult to generalize about it without making people uncomfortable, without leaving someone out, without violating someone's right to be different. Nevertheless, with ADD people, there are some generalities I can outline. The big generality is, simply, sex with (and for) an ADD person requires some understanding, or it's destined to cause frustration and dissatisfaction. This means that the ability to communicate verbally is essential to let personal needs and wants be known.

As importantly, from foreplay to location, variety is often the key to sex with an ADD person. Remember, ADD people tend to get easily bored with the same thing. Fortunately, at least for them, ADD people usually also have a willingness to experiment, to have sex in different ways in different settings.

An ADD person can get a lot out of foreplay if the individuals are comfortable with sex at all and if they mutually like each other and want each other physically. Because of the tension-relieving nature of sex, foreplay often acts as a reminder of pleasures to come. And usually, there's not a problem concentrating on it, providing you keep it varied, and it's not prolonged. This is true even when the relationship is full of fighting and conflict.

119

Sex makes people feel that they have some control: "Here's a person I care about, and I have a guaranteed outcome."

If the couple is not in tune with one another, loving and liking each other, the guaranteed outcome will not be there. A person with ADD can then be rejecting, feeling intruded upon by the partner's sexual desires or blaming the partner for the problems they are having. It's important that the partner accept no more than half the responsibility for the lack of fulfillment.

But, even with loving, caring couples, it's important to remember the ADD person's extreme sensitivity to pleasure and pain and the way the person feels things strongly, and act accordingly. This characteristic can be used to advantage, if you do it right, and can lead to the greatest pleasure two people can share.

Some practical tips: One ADD person I know likes the light touch of fingernails drawn across her skin, but not too much in one place. Another likes being stroked with an ice cube, and another likes being licked (try honey or chocolate)—but, again never too long in one place.

Variation in sexual position follows the same rule of thumb: Anything goes that will keep interest heightened. (Obviously the variation must be acceptable to both partners or not pursued at the expense of one.) Oral sex can fill the need for diversity but it is imperative that good hygiene be followed. Remember, all of the senses of a person with ADD are heightened. If his or her sense of smell or taste is offended, the desire for intimacy is squelched.

Because of the ADD person's sensitivity to pain, men must be especially mindful of finding comfortable positions for intercourse with an ADD female. Good communication and willingness to be flexible are essential here. ADD persons of either sex will generally experience the pressure of weight on top of them as more uncomfortable than non-ADD folks, so they may resist having the partner on top during intercourse. The key is understanding and the willingness to find positions that feel good to both participants.

Vary the location and environment for sex. Don't just have it in the bedroom, but try the living room or back seat of the car. Try it in the swimming pool. Try turning off the air conditioner to build up a sweat. Switch from cotton sheets to satin sheets in the summer and flannel sheets in the winter. Remember, variety is the key for most ADD adults.

▶ Sexual Repression

There are exceptions, however, to this rule. After all, comfort with experimentation depends on how a person was trained about sex, whether they were raised with a sense of safety about it. Without such an upbringing, an ADD person may want no variability. Experimentation and prolonged sexual expression may seem too dangerous. Having sex the same way all the time may make him or her feel safe. Otherwise, he or she will make every effort to avoid sex—and exhibit the rigidity that some associate with Attention Deficit Disorder. There will be a tendency to make sex mechanical.

▶ When You're the Significant Other

Sounds like I'm talking about sex as a one-way street? Everything you can do for your ADD mate, sure, but what about you? It doesn't hurt to satisfy your mate's special needs, but what about yours? As with any intimate relationship without ADD, it's imperative that both participants are satisfied: no losers. Communication and consensus are the keys to making this happen.

There's nothing wrong with saying, "It's my turn now." One day, do it his way, the next, try it yours. Let your partner know what you like and ask. Don't demand, whine, or scold. Remember, most ADD people like humor, so it may do you

121

well to add some instead of taking the sex game too seriously. Teasingly, you might say, "Watch out! I'll get you when you're least expecting it . . . okay, not really. But let's play, huh?" It will be the lighthearted tone in your voice that will entice your lover.

Remember, the vulnerable feelings of an ADD person are soothed by reassurances that you won't hurt her. Better you learn to back off for a while than ruin the whole thing by impatiently trying to force sex. Say, "I'll stop if you want me to, but will you bring me to climax?" It's important that the ADD person not leave you hanging, so communicate your needs.

Consensus is a couple's best friend, not compromise. In the latter, neither gets what he wants. In consensus, together you find an alternative that pleases both. Don't give in and set yourself up as a loser. Don't get impatient because you are having trouble finding the solution. Say, "I know we'll find what is good for both of us. I love you."

If your partner will not work with you, you may need to be very clear that you can't do it all yourself. Sex is one area in which you cannot succeed alone, and going outside the partnership for sexual satisfaction is questionable. It's better to face the fact that there is an unwillingness to work with you on sexual issues and get on with your life. Seek marriage counseling and be willing to call it quits if the willingness to try has vanished.

It is important to distinguish between a willingness to try and an ability to succeed. If you hear "I'm sorry," then you at least know you are being considered. You may be expected to be told you are important and lovable, which means your partner is taking responsibility for his part in this. ADD or not, no partner gets a free ride. Understanding, yes. A free ride, no.

▶ Common Questions about Intimacy

> ▶ **My wife has trouble maintaining eye contact in a conversation with me, keeps fiddling with things, and**

gets up and moves around instead of paying attention to me. Is she bored with me or could it be caused by ADD?

It could be ADD and it might not be. A good diagnostic workup is essential to determine whether it is or not.

But, in an intimate relationship, ADD or not, you need to work at good communication. Ask your wife how she is feeling. Ask her whether it would be easier for her to talk with you in short segments or while she's walking around.

Check to see what the style of your conversation is. Do you lecture, scold, go on and on, talk only about yourself, or monopolize the conversation?

▶ **I feel hurt because of her behavior. What can I do to feel better?**

Getting your feelings hurt is a great way to wreck a relationship. It puts responsibility for how you feel on the other person. Sounds like something you learned from your own past.

To remedy the situation, do two basic things:

▶ Look at your own expectations to see what it is you think your wife ought to be doing for you. Then do it yourself.

▶ Ask your wife whether she intended to hurt you with her behavior. She'll probably look utterly amazed and say, "No."

▶ **What can I do to make the situation better?**

Ask your wife to join you at a specific time and place, on a regular basis, so you can share some conversation and caring. Sometimes do what she suggests and sometimes

123

you take the lead. A good marriage, with or without ADD, takes time and attention but the labor is worth it. Don't hesitate to work with a marriage counselor if things don't get a lot better.

► **My husband, who has ADD, might be called the one-minute lover. I'm not making fun of him; it's just true. He has no need for foreplay, especially anything I might need or prefer. I need more—more intimacy, more of everything. What can I do?**

Find a neutral time, not when you are already in bed, to talk about the situation. Start with something positive like how much you care about him and would like making love with him.

Determine whether he has gotten into a bad habit of being thoughtless about you or whether he is truly suffering from a condition called premature ejaculation. A marriage counselor or sex therapist can help you with the latter. You and he can do a lot about the thoughtlessness.

Then, ask for his help. Take small steps, asking for a little fondling at first. Tell him how important it is to you. Be careful not to blame, criticize, or scold him about his lovemaking. But do make your point that you are important and want to have fun, too.

Do not necessarily expect to climax at the same time. If he has already come, ask him to continue to make love to you until you do. Or turn it around and ask him to make love to you first.

Above all, do not make the remediation of the problem too serious. Add some fun along with a full measure of sensitivity and enjoy one another.

▶ **My partner wants to talk and talk and talk about sex: What she prefers, what made her feel good last night, and what she wants to try next. Is this because of her ADD? Just how much conversation about sex is necessary because of ADD and how much is due to other factors? Frankly, I find most of it boring.**

Although excessive talking is sometimes a symptom of ADD, it may or may not be due to her brain wiring. It could be nervousness or anxiety or just a problem with compulsive talking.

Some talk about your needs and hers seems indicated here if only for the sake of comfort. Do be sensitive, and for heaven's sake don't tell her you're bored. Make an "I statement," such as "I'm having trouble concentrating while you're talking. Would you tell me how the talking helps you? I'd really like to understand." Then listen.

She may be afraid because of past experience that her needs will be overlooked. Try to assure her that you want her to get what she wants and that you will work on it a little at a time. Be sure to ask her if she's pleased with whatever you do.

▶ **I'm a hugger, toucher, and feeler. It's just the way I am. I'm married to an ADD person who really doesn't like to be touched, at least not in the way I like to touch. What can we do? How can one of us not lose in this situation? Are we doomed for frustration or divorce?**

Since you are the one who likes to be touched, let her do the touching of you rather than vice versa. I wonder if you haven't been touching her as a way to initiate sex, which turns her off. Ask for what you want and you may have a deal.

The real trick in intimacy is to have no losers. there is always a loser if force or coercion is used. Therefore, you two must find ways to be together that satisfy both of you. To accomplish this, talk, experiment, and try some soothing oils. Be sure with your ADD wife that you touch her gently and firmly and don't stay in one place very long. No tickling.

► **I have ADD, and it takes me a long time to reach orgasm. I keep getting distracted, and my partner eventually gets bored. What's the solution?**

Taking a long time to reach orgasm may not be the result of ADD. Neither is your distractibility. First, get a physical with your gynecologist. Then, if all is okay, look for causative factors in what you were taught about sex and what your previous sexual experiences may have been. If you were mistreated or were sexually abused, you would have learned to distract yourself as a psychological protection. It's hard to turn your awareness back on, even though it's now safe. Counseling offers a lot of good help for this kind of problem. Finally, check to be sure you are attracted to your partner.

When I sleep, I like to be tucked under the covers and hold my wife like a pillow. She hates it and says it feels like she's being suffocated. Yet I have a hard time falling asleep without it. What can I do?

Better get yourself a real pillow to hug.

Occasionally embracing your wife would probably feel good to her. But using her like a pillow for comfort is asking too much of her. Slowly wean yourself away from the habit.

► **My wife, who is ADD, is really adamant when she talks about what she likes sexually. Yet it seems that what she likes changes constantly. I get confused. What does she *really* like?**

Variation.

▶ **If I suggest sexual experimentation, my husband, who has ADD, objects. But if he suggests it, then it's okay. Is this because he has ADD, or is he just selfish?**

One of the characteristics of people with ADD is a desire to be in control of things that affect them. Is it any wonder, since their neurology put them at a disadvantage early on? But you count too. So, tell him you understand his need but you want to cut a deal, share and share alike. Mentally healthy people with ADD are very willing to share. If he is not, then it's not the ADD that is making him controlling; it's an emotional problem and you need to be firm that he really can't have only his way.

◄ı◄ı◄|12|►ı►ı►

When You Work with an ADD Person

▼

*H*aving become familiar with Attention Deficit Disorder, it is quite possible that you now see signs of it in people with whom you work. Or, worse yet, you think your boss demonstrates characteristics of ADD. But you can't go up to a co-worker or your boss and say, "I think you are ADD."

Sure, when you came for the job interview and met your new co-workers, there were no signs. But day in and day out, working with someone with untreated ADD has led to frustration, lost motivation, and feelings of resentment over having to do more than your fair share. And the worst part is that, unlike at home where you can blow off steam with your spouse, child, or parent, on the job you have to deal with the problem and your feelings about it without openly acknowledging that they even exist. *You* have to take responsibility for managing their ADD.

The following common questions and their answers will help you learn what you can do to make life easier on the job when you work with or for someone who has ADD but is not taking responsibility for it. These examples are taken from real life situations with real people who have either been diagnosed to have

ADD or who believe they are working with someone with undi-agnosed ADD.

▶ **My boss agrees to my plans one day and the next day tells me he never said "yes." How can he not remember what he said?**

Typical of ADD is a phenomenon in which the person says "yes" automatically, trying to be the good guy. Actually, when the "yes" is spoken, it may not be attached to a request in his mind. So, unbeknownst to you, your question never really got through.

▶ **My co-worker has all sorts of ideas but doesn't follow through on any of them. Is she just irresponsible?**

Could be. Might not be. Could be that her intent is to follow through but she gets distracted. She could be trying to be a good guy also, agreeing to develop much more than she can handle and getting lost in the aftermath.

To be honest with you, most people who appear irresponsible are trying the best they can. There could be other learning disabilities or emotional problems that are getting in the way of the completion of their objectives.

To protect yourself, don't depend on her for something you need done. Listen to her ideas but don't spend time putting work into them until she gets her ability to complete things under control.

▶ **My boss jumps from one topic to the next without resolving any of them. Business meetings seem pointless, but I can't refuse to attend. What can I do?**

▶ You can take a pad and do your own work during the meeting.

130

▶ From time to time you can suggest to your boss that you skip a meeting to complete a project.

▶ You can ask pointed questions during the meeting so that you get what you need out of it.

▶ You can listen to the topics your boss raises during the meeting, identify the ones that pertain directly to you, and, after the meeting, go to the people from whom you need input and get it personally rather than in the group. If you need further input from your boss, you might try getting it in writing.

▶ **Whenever I have something long or complicated to explain to my boss, he doesn't seem to be able to focus on what I'm saying. How can I communicate with him more effectively?**

Try putting what you have to say in written form. Maybe even outline it. Give him direct written questions to answer, preferably with "yes" or "no" answers.

If you talk with him, give him one question at a time. Get the answer to that one before going on to the next question. Don't expect to have lengthy conversations. Rather, touch base with him several times during the day so that your encounters are in small segments.

▶ **A co-worker doesn't keep her commitments, and I'm beginning to feel I can't trust her. But she is so likable, and I don't want to just give up on her. What can I do?**

Separate your work needs from your personal feelings. You can enjoy her as a person even though you do not depend on her. For heaven's sake, don't expect her to come through. She apparently isn't able at this time. So, if you expect follow-through on commitments, you're only setting yourself up for disappointment.

Also, give her permission to tell you "no" when you do

131

ask her to do something. She may be succumbing to the good guy syndrome.

► **My boss can't seem to remember a production schedule he has worked with for years. Is he just not trying?**

It's possible he doesn't care and isn't trying but not likely. After all, it is his living also that's in jeopardy.

Unless he has a chemical abuse problem, he probably simply does not think about schedules, especially if he is a creative type of person. He may also get distracted by all sorts of issues that emerge in the daily running of a business or by his own ideas.

Your best bet to remedy the problem is to post a clear schedule, bring his attention to it regularly, and take as much personal responsibility as you can manage to keep up with it. Use his skills where they do shine. Some people just plain don't do well with schedules.

► **My boss is rigid and gets very upset if I deviate one little bit from the schedule he insists we use.**

Here's the flip side of the above coin. This boss has compensated for his deficits by rigidly adhering to a schedule or has the highly structured form of ADD (see appendices). The reason is that, if he gets off schedule a little bit, he'll get off of it a lot. There tends to be no middle ground with people who are ADD.

► **The guy I work with just seems to bounce around. He has so much energy that he's like a puppy. How can I calm him down?**

There may be very little that you can do to calm him down. Though most people who have Attention Deficit Disorder have increased motor activity, only some have hyperactivity that is as noticeable as your co-worker's.

The best you can do is to talk and move smoothly and soothingly. Your manner can calm him down a little. You may be able to affect him if you simply talk in a slower, soothing manner. Lower your voice. Try it.

▶ **Everyone likes our P.R. (public relations) director because she's so friendly and cheerful. But she just doesn't do well at her work. She's always distracted. I'm the one who has to follow through for her, but if I criticize her, I'm viewed as the bad guy. Is there any way to win in this situation?**

Be very straightforward with her, first of all. She needs to do something about her lack of follow-through. Tell her you have a problem because she doesn't produce on time, and tell her what you're going to do about it. Say, "I got into a real bind yesterday because your material wasn't ready. I know you're doing the best you can, and I like you a lot, but I can't run short again next week. Is there anything I can do to help you?" Offer help, but don't set yourself up as a judge or criticize her.

If there continues to be a problem, ask her to join you for a discussion with your boss to work out a solution. That way you don't have to be the bad guy and you can get what you need.

If you are empathic with her, you may be amazed at how she may confide her fears and problems to you, considering you her good friend.

▶ **I hired a woman I thought was wonderful but she can't ever finish what she starts. My co-workers expect me to handle the work—she's my employee, after all. But if I criticize her work at all, she says I'm picking on her. What can I say to make things better? What are my options?**

How you bring her attention to inadequacies is impor-

133

tant. If you tell her what's wrong without telling her how to fix it, she will feel helpless. After all, if she could have done it right in the first place, she would have. Instead, point out what you like or find acceptable in her work. Do this in a matter-of-fact way. Then show her how to apply that to something else she is doing.

Be sure to give her small assignments that are very specific. You may be giving her too much at one time so she can't focus. Give her breaking points in the work so she can naturally change her focus of attention rather than having it happen to her. What I'm talking about is providing more structure. (The armed services do it effectively. Take note.)

If your employee has an attitude problem, you can mention it to her, asking whether something is bothering her personally that she has been unable to leave at home.

Then, remember, if you hired her, you can fire her. You can do it humanely by taking responsibility. Say, "I made a mistake and hired you to do something that doesn't fit your capabilities. The job is not getting done, and you aren't getting the satisfaction of going a job well," You may want to counsel her with regard to a job that would better suit her. You may also want to mention to her that you feel she may have an attention problem that could be helped. Tell her you believe she is doing the best she can do and must be frustrated, but that help is available. Then refer her on to a counselor or support group that works with ADD *and* emotional problems.

If she still insists you are picking on her, say, "I'm sorry you feel that way, but it seems I can't do anything to change your mind." Then back off.

▶ **The wife of one of my best employees is a saleswoman. He is often late to functions, saying, "My wife** just can't get anywhere on time." What could be the problem? What can he do to correct it?

There are many reasons people are late. ADD is one, but by no means the only one. It could be her way of asserting her power in the relationship. (He wants her to be on time, so she gets to him by not being on time.) It could be an expression of the fact that she doesn't want to go.

What he can do to correct it is to take responsibility for getting himself to the function on time. He can come ahead and she can join him later. How he works that out with her is his business. You just keep the limit in place that you expect him on time and don't let him use his wife as an excuse.

► **My boss changes his mind about our plans all the time. He seems to jump from one idea to another. It causes me to make a lot of false starts, wastes a lot of my time, and makes me feel frustrated. How should I talk with him about this, and will it do any good?**

Go to him and say you appreciate the many ideas he has. Say, "But, I'm the kind of person who needs to follow through on ideas, and that's why you hired me. I need you to choose which idea you want me to work on to completion." Say it in a firm, slightly serious but warm manner. This lets him know you mean business but are not being critical.

When he again starts spewing off new ideas, make a list of them, taking the list to him along with a list of the projects you are already involved with. Ask him to set priorities. Say, warmly and firmly, "Remember, I need to feel good about finishing something." That way the burden is placed on him with regard to how you spend your time.

Most creative people, with or without ADD, appreciate

135

having someone like you around. Your boss needs you desperately but just doesn't know how to use you. Help him learn.

If he is unwilling to work with you or fails to be nice about it, then look for another job.

▶ **One week my boss is incredibly excited about a project, demanding I act on it right away; the next week she's forgotten about it. Should I just ignore her fits of enthusiasm in the first place? Do you suppose I might be fired if I do?**

Gently point out a specific situation to her saying, "I was in the middle of Project A when you asked me to start work on Project B, which you were very excited about at the time. Now, you have dismissed Project B. I'm confused. I need your help. I need to stick to one project until it is done or, if we switch gears, stay switched. What do you want me to do?"

You will be talking to the reasoning part of your boss, not the emotional part (from which the new ideas come) and are likely to get a good, straightforward response as long as you don't sound critical.

Then ask her what she wants you to do if she again enthusiastically comes to you with a new idea. On her rational, reasoning mode, she will tell you what she needs. Then do it, and don't worry about getting fired.

▶ **I feel like I'm working with a toddler sometimes. My co-worker has the shortest attention span I've ever seen. She'll stop talking in the middle of her own sentences or walk away in the middle of mine. What's the matter with her, and what can I do?**

She certainly changes the focus of her attention frequently. It could be caused by any number of things including emotional problems, ADD, a seizure disorder, or some other organic problem. But it could also be that she's incredibly creative. Don't expect to diagnose it yourself.

What you can do is:

▶ Not take it personally.

▶ Keep your own conversations with her short. If she still walks away, go to her and ask whether she had a problem with what you were saying so you get some clarification for yourself. Tell her you need to hear the *end* of her sentence.

▶ Accept her as she is and don't expect more than what she can give.

▶ **My boss only seems to want to dream and make big plans. I'm beginning to think he does this because of the excitement he gets out of it. Could that be?**

Sure could. There is a high (an adrenaline rush) that comes from the making of big plans. Some people get it from just having a wonderful idea. The feeling that comes from the high is so good that the person tends to want to feel it again and again. Once the feeling has passed, there is little interest in continuing to develop the plan. After all, it's pretty hard to get a rush from following up on mundane details. Sometimes the person doesn't know *how* to follow up.

▶ **Is there any future for me in a job where there's no follow-through by my boss on his dreams? What can I do to change things?**

Being in a dependent position in relation to a dreamer is risky unless that person is enough in touch with reality to appreciate what you bring to the situation. Dreamers need clear-minded thinkers and doers who can take

137

responsibility to manifest their dreams. Your future depends upon your boss appreciating what you have to offer and giving you the power to do your job. That includes allowing you to set limits on him, such as saying, "No, we're not going to act on your new dream until we have completed work on the current dream project."

▶ **My boss comes into my office and demands I clean up my desk. He says no one could possibly do a good job with so much confusion. I know exactly where everything is and can find what I need when I need it—and quickly. Why can't he leave my desk alone?**

You boss is assuming that because he is bothered by clutter on his desk, that you would be too. Empathize with him, saying, "I realize the shape my desk is in would make you feel confused, but my mind works differently and I do better this way." Then reassure him, saying, "I'll take responsibility to get my work done. Feel free to criticize me on those grounds but leave my desk alone." It won't hurt to add a bit of humor to these statements.

If he comes in again and says something, jokingly say, "Out of here."

▶ **Why would someone not do any of the things necessary to get a big bonus based on the completion of jobs when he is immensely talented and seems to like what he is doing?**

It all depends on what those things are that he has to do to get the bonus. His talent may simply lie in other areas and he may prefer not to do them. Money is not the primary reward for many creative people. The chance to do what they like to do may be more important.

▶ **My office mate can't seem to remember the promises he makes me. Then he acts like a little kid who should** just be excused every time. Does he just do that to play me along, never intending to keep his promises in the first place? What's his problem?

First of all, your office mate probably learned early in life that more was expected of him than he could manage to do (not uncommon with people with ADD). He also learned that if he promised he'd do something, his parents or teachers went easier on him. Such promises bought him time to try to figure out some way to please these important people. You see, all children desperately want to please the adults around them.

Unfortunately, no one realized that more was being expected than the little child could produce (also a common factor in ADD because the ability to produce results lags behind the general intelligence and capability of the child).

Then, to add insult to injury, your office mate was taught to say, "I'm sorry," whether he was really sorry or not. Unfortunately, this is common in our culture. It is the way he learned to get people off his back when he failed to follow through on something.

Your job is to tell him that you are more interested in his only committing to do what he knows he is willing to do, that you will like him even if he says "no" to you, and that you are more interested in problem solving when something isn't completed than hearing, "I'm sorry." Say, "Let's see what the problem is and figure out how to solve it. I know you care."

▶ My boss just doesn't listen to me, because I'm telling him things he doesn't want to hear. But I'm the office bookkeeper and most of what I have to tell him isn't good news. What can I do?

▶ Keep your sense of humor.

139

► Realize that he is running away from things that cause him anxiety.

► Rather than telling him the problem first, which raises his anxiety level, tell him something he can do to fix the problem.

► A lot depends on how close he will let you get to his feelings. If your relationship warrants it, you can get right up in his face and talk turkey to him, confronting him. But you have to have someone's trust to do that.

► Realize the limits of your power. You are the employee and he's the boss. If he continues to run, he's committing business suicide and you cannot take the responsibility to stop him. You can only try to help him.

► Be protective of yourself if you realize the company may be going under, and start looking for other opportunities.

► **Our sales manager can't seem to organize his own time. I see this in other sales reps also, so I'm not sure I'll do much better if I fire him. Besides, he makes good sales. Any suggestions?**

There is a higher than average number of people with ADD who are drawn to sales positions, often doing very well. However, organization is often not their strong suit (though some have mastered the problem by being extremely organized.)

Keep paperwork to a minimum. Try providing simple, clearly structured report sheets. Have the person take part in the development of the reporting form. As you see from the samples in Chapter 9, different people with ADD handle their structuring differently. Be flexible.

If no choice is available, break the task into small segments, so, rather than doing all the reports on Friday, have him do them daily. (Don't be surprised, though, to discover that when he is on the road, he'll avoid doing the reports until the last minute. Many of us tend to have an aversion to doing what is very hard, so we put it off.)

Empathize with your errant salesperson and be grateful for what you do have.

Consider hiring a clerk so the salesperson only has to collect raw data that someone else puts in boxes. Then, the salesperson can go out and sell more to pay for the clerk.

▶ **My business partner never does what he says he is going to do. But if I get irritated with him, he just falls apart. Why is he like this?**

He probably has a long history of people getting mad at him for not producing what he is supposed to produce. And, if he's a typical ADD person, he has a great need (who among us doesn't?) to be liked. So he falls apart because he feels awful.

Now, I'm going to pin you to the wall. Why do you feel irritated? We can observe a problem without getting emotionally upset, unless there is something for us to learn from the situation about ourselves. Many folks, however, tend to put the responsibility for their feelings on others.

Ask yourself, "When else in my life have I been in a situation in which someone has let me down, saying they would do something and then not following through?" You may remember when your dad said he's go to your ballgame to watch you play. You told all the kids he was coming and he never showed up. PAIN! Though your irritation may come from a less painful memory, there will be something for you to learn. His lack of follow-through may cause you to have to do more work or compromise your safety or security.

Knowing the cause of your irritation can help you remove it from your conversation with your partner. Then you can talk in matter-of-fact, non-critical business terms that will get to the real issues rather than emotional issues.

Lay out the tangible business needs you have, ask your partner to commit to only what he is willing and able to do. (Many people with ADD want to produce more than they are actually able to produce.)

Your partner must get beyond his part of this problem so you can count on him to be trustworthy. Otherwise, it is not wise to be in a partnership that can compromise your security.

On occasion, it may be worthwhile to stay in the partnership, working behind the scenes to do both your work and what your partner promises to do, if you are getting something else of value from him, such as financial backing. Just know the price you are paying for the backing and don't expect more.

► **I know my boss is intelligent, but sometimes he doesn't act like it. He can't seem to focus on giving me work to do in an efficient manner so I come off looking bad. What can I do to protect myself from looking bad?**

Don't expect your boss to do the organizing. You do it. No matter how intelligent your boss, you may be a much better organizer. Or work with him to get organized.

▶ Another manager in our department has terrible work habits but keeps getting awards for innovative ideas. But she never follows through on them, and her paperwork is a mess. I try very hard and have good work habits but get overlooked. Why does upper management notice her all the time? What can I do to get noticed?

Apparently upper management hasn't caught on to the fact that she doesn't follow through. Patience, my dear. Sooner or later, they will realize the problem unless they value ideas without follow-through.

To get noticed, you may need to call their attention to a completed project. Blow your own horn. Were you by any chance taught that that was not the thing to do to be polite? Or worse yet, maybe it wasn't even safe for you in your family to be noticed. Work on these issues within yourself so you can show your stuff off.

Finally, you may, after some patience, decide that there is not a good fit between you and upper management. At that point, get another job where you and your skills will be valued.

Epilogue

▼

*P*eople who are ADD have been drawn to me like bears to honey. I, in turn, love the wonderful characteristics that are part of some of the sweetest, most sensitive people in the world. I married a person who is ADD, though I didn't realize it at the time. I reared at least one son who is ADD. My personal friends are disproportionately weighted in that direction. The people I have connected with through radio, television, and public appearances frequently have had more than their fair share of ADD attributes, and my private practice brought me in touch with many others with whom I have been able to work effectively. And finally, I, too, know that I am ADD.

I began to wonder one day why, or how, this magnetism between me and so many ADD persons had developed. The answer, I believe, lies in characteristics we share.

I am very sensitive and feel things deeply. I am creative by nature and in my approach to problems. I am learning disabled, as are many people who are ADD, so I know the feelings of lost potential first hand. I'm empathic with regard to the feelings of others. I get bored easily, can't sit still, and don't organize well—at least as judged by most people. All these traits I share with people who have ADD brain wiring.

145

But I have also been highly socialized and have learned a lot of self-discipline. Because of this I can stay focused on a task for a long period of time, though I feel restless inside. I am patient and soothing and become more so when I am around someone who is scattered, stressed, or out of control. I've learned to use my ADD to my advantage.

I truly admire the characteristics displayed by those of us who are ADD; I also feel the pain. Communicating this understanding builds an instant bond between myself and others who are ADD. I also have the skills to help others heal their pain, as I have done with much of mine, so that we can grow beyond the difficulties encountered in a non-ADD culture. I have never met a more grateful group of people.

People with ADD tend to wear their emotions on their sleeves. Holding few secrets, we display our feelings and thoughts to the world. We know what it's like to be hurt, and because we crave acceptance and understanding, we often readily accord it to others. We are easier to deal with than people who do things because they *should* rather than from the depths of their hearts. No pretense here.

In my dealing with ADD, I've also learned to look at it in another way—to look at what I'm tempted to call its advantages. For example, it's difficult to fool people with ADD. We look past surface appearances and facades to the core of people and issues and evaluate them with down-to-earth standards. We may see the truth even when another person denies it. We tend to be good networkers, because we see so many relationships between people and things.

Also, because we don't suffer from the boundary isolation that "normal" people are afflicted with, we are able to put new projects together readily. We can cross disciplines or skill areas, drawing from what attracts our attention. Without the boundaries that confine non-ADD people, we focus on relationships found between disciplines. Because we can so easily switch our attention from one thing to another, we do not get in a rut.

Our sometimes chaotic perception makes us original, flipping from one train of thought to another, with a marvelous sense of humor. We don't miss a cue. At the best of times, we are fun to go places with because we see things other people don't see. We are observers par excellence. If you've lost something, call your nearest ADD friend. We are more likely to find it than the average person. Our observatory power is why we make good salespeople, broadcasters, creative people, and entrepreneurs.

The wealth of talent and goodness possessed by people with ADD tends to be ignored. Creative and spontaneous, these often-misunderstood folks may be one of the great unrecognized treasures of our land. We are a national resource that can be tapped. All it will take is understanding, some adjustments in the educational process to better fit our style of learning, and awareness on the part of parents so that they can adjust their parenting styles. Children who are ADD can be taught to adjust to a non-ADD culture, speak out about it, and as they mature, put themselves in learning and work environments that will use their talents and gifts effectively. ADD, really, is as much of an asset as a liability.

The "disorder," as it is called, provides people with a different way of looking at the world and creates the need for a different way of learning. Trying to fit ADD people into the non-ADD world order causes problems for both the system and the ADD person. Try pulling a fish out of the water demanding that it learn to live in the world of air. Send it to flying school and watch what happens.

ADD people usually benefit from an opportunity to move around, learn by doing, do projects in short segments, organize in their own ways, and are creative in their approach to tasks. If an ADD person is told the desired outcome and is allowed to develop in his or her own way toward the arrival of that outcome, the project is more likely to succeed.

But try to squeeze us into a stereotypical pattern and there is likely to be a lot of hollering and wasted energy. So concentrate on the intent of the project or activity. Specify the desired outcome. This is critical when working with someone who is ADD.

Most importantly—throw the rule book aside! Let the ADD person develop his own path and his own timetable. If you do this, you are likely to get an A-1 job out of the ADD person.

The loss of potential through underachievement, drug and alcohol abuse, and delinquent behavior caused by untreated ADD is a crime of its own. It costs taxpayers millions of dollars every year, wrecks the lives of innocent people, breaks up marriages, and carves a path of destruction and pain for the victims and their family members.

Yet those losses needn't occur. ADD can be recognized at an early age—or any time thereafter. Adults with ADD can turn their lives around. Through training and education we can right previous wrongs, breaking the cycle of devastation that has been passed from generation to generation.

Though I'm not much of an activist or placard carrier, I am campaigning for awareness of this very workable difference, previously called a condition or disorder. Now I realize ADD is a civil rights issue, not a disability. Please join me—for yourself, your loved ones, and your friends.

▶ A Few Last Questions About ADD

▶ What are the advantages to having ADD?

Advantages to having ADD include creativity, an ease in sharing thoughts and feelings, and a tendency to offer acceptance and understanding to others. People with ADD have a high degree of sensitivity and empathy.

We do not tend to be "should" people but do what we feel. We can look through facades and see people and issues clearly, so we are more truthful than many others. We do not have boundary isolation, i.e., we do not limit ourselves to one area, but rather see the similarities between things. So we are good at interdisciplinary and cross-disciplinary skills. We see processes and patterns where others see details and minutiae. We are very intense when very interested in something.

▶ **Aren't there other ways to get these traits?**

Sure. Not only is not every person with ADD necessarily creative, but not all creative people have ADD. There are many reasons why each of the traits develops in different people. It's just that people with ADD tend to have them as a kind of side effect of the way we're wired.

▶ **What is boundary isolation?**

It is a kind of territoriality on a mental or emotional level. Our culture tends to be very territorial. One professional doesn't want anyone schooled outside of that profession to be able to ply the skills identified as belonging to that profession. Labels are attached to the categories regardless of the similarities in the way they may function.

In boundary diffusion, the opposite is true. Similarities in function are what is important. The category in which the skill belongs is irrelevant.

For example, the best training I ever received for counseling people came from my graduate work in anthropology, where I learned a research method called "participant observation." But rather than applying it to anthropology, I became aware that it was exactly what happens in counseling when the therapist affects the client(s) by his or her presence. So I applied what I learned across disciplines. Then I applied it to parenting, managing my office staff, etc. And it doesn't matter to me that participant observation is generally considered to be a tool of anthropologists; it is still useful.

This is what happens in boundary diffusion.

APPENDICES

If You Think You May Be ADD, Read On

▼

*A*ttention Deficit Disorder is one of those "conditions" that often goes unrecognized as the culprit beneath other problems that plague a person in the growing years. It is not unusual in adolescence for people with ADD to self-medicate with drugs and alcohol, to do poorly in school even though bright. "You could do better if you'd just try," is a common complaint leveled at an ADD person, who comes to believe that, indeed, he or she ought to be able to pay attention to meaningless material and produce in ways that don't fit.

Active, creative, sensitive, restless, sometimes explosive, requiring variability in all areas of life, the person with ADD can be channeled to find a place in adult life that fits. But all too often the criticisms and abuse of early years leave their mark on the self-confidence and self-esteem of the adult. The ADD adult *believes* himself/herself to be of lesser stock or inferior quality than peers because of a condition that makes its mark in terms of the way the person experiences the world.

Diagnostic criteria for ADD include:

A history (often undiagnosed) of ADD must be present in childhood. (A hyper kid, he or she talked too much, bounced around the classroom, tended to get in more trouble than other kids for small things, and didn't seem to learn from experience because he or she continually did things over and over. This kid didn't like school much and often was criticized and even abused because of problems concentrating, staying on task, and sitting still.)

Also there must be both attention and motor problems in the adult. Typically, these show up in difficulty completing a task if not particularly interested in it. (A well socialized person will complete the task but inwardly will need to use an inordinate amount of effort to do so.) Often this criterion is used as a criticism, "You could do it if you wanted to." Those who do not have ADD can do it even if they don't want to, but an ADD person is much more likely to be distracted if he is not interested in the task at hand.

Difficulty in maintaining concentration in conversation with others, particularly in groups, is prevalent. Listening to verbal reports, lectures, and meetings may be hard for the ADD person, especially if the speaker talks in a monotone or is not demonstrative.

ADD motor behavior takes three forms in adulthood. The first behavior, motor restlessness, can be expressed as an inability to relax unless fatigued. A person might seem to be, until he sits or lies down—then he is likely to go to sleep or "blob out" couch potato style in front of the TV. The restlessness may be subtle with the shifting of weight, lots of trips to the water cooler, or movement disguised as involvement in many activities. These forms are more apparent when a person has been well socialized and is trying very hard to do what is "right."

Fidgeting is the second form of motor compromise. This includes finger and toe tapping, sometimes disguised by the subtle depression of the appendage so that no one really notices. Leg swinging, seat shifting, and general continuous motion are apparent often.

Some ADD adults are underactive, staying very still as if

they've been hypnotized—for example, while they're sitting at a computer.

Other characteristic ADD attributes in adulthood include: poor impulse control; wide mood variation; short or excessive temper and/or irritability; poor linear organization of external tasks, with difficulty completing tasks; high sensitivity with subsequent high reactivity levels; and low stress tolerance.

People with poor impulse control have difficulty in delaying gratification, are unable to anticipate consequences, and say things on the spur of the moment. They frequently act without thinking. I've often been told by ADD people that "if I don't do something immediately, I'll never get it done because I'll get distracted." Breaking into a conversation, buying impulsively, drinking impulsively, and other similar behaviors often bring severe repercussions and certainly can disrupt social relationships.

Mood variability includes feeling very, very good and very, very bad, often within a short period of time. However, the mood changes are environmentally related. The person with ADD also gets over the downs quickly, especially if the outside situation rights itself.

Poor organization with a difficulty completing external tasks occurs as the ADD person jumps from one thing to another. Some ADD people have a good ability to structure their work but may still have problems in actually following the structure they themselves have created. It is not unusual for a person with ADD to live in a state of mental and physical clutter, and it is important to not overload the person with too much new input too quickly. Much difficulty with organization is due to a lack of early training during youth that will fit natural, internal organization styles.

High levels of sensitivity with low stress tolerance and overreactivity looks like "emotional thin skin." Actually, when you consider the problems in screening out stimuli, the ADD person is reacting appropriately to their screening mechanism. Their screening mechanism is just a lot more sensitive than that of people without ADD. So, ADD people are easily flustered, feel hassled, tense, or uptight. Others think we make mountains out of molehills.

People with ADD like vibration, rock and roll, drums, soothing partners, and freedom of motion. When the condition is understood and guilt over past and present inabilities to "control" ourselves is let go, an ADD person can make adjustments that allow for a perfectly happy life in which his or her attributes are seen as assets rather than liabilities.

Official Diagnosis of
ADD in Adults

▼

► **American Psychiatric Association
Diagnostic and Statistical Manual**

The Diagnostic and Statistical Manual (DSM) published by the American Psychiatric Association contains definitions and codes for psychiatric conditions, including Attention Deficit Disorder. The information is used to communicate between physicians and other medical personnel, insurance companies, and anyone involved with the treatment of the person diagnosed to have a condition included in the book.

Often the definition impacts who is identified as having a condition and therefore who gets treated; how he is treated; and how much money the person will pay out-of-pocket for the treatment. Insurance companies, agencies, and programs (such as the rehabilitation commissions) of the various states will set their parameters for treatment based on what is included under the categories of the DSM.

In 1980, Attention Deficit Disorder in Adults made its debut in DSM-III. It was listed in the section on "Disorders Usually First Evident in Infancy, Childhood or Adolescence." The disorder was called Attention Deficit Disorder, Residual Type, and given a code of 314.80.

*Diagnostic criteria for Attention Deficit Disorder,
Residual Type*

A. The individual once met the criteria for Attention Deficit Disorder with Hyperactivity.

This information may come from the individual or from others, such as family members.

B. Signs of hyperactivity are no longer present, but other signs of the illness have persisted to the present without periods of remission, as evidenced by signs of both attention deficits and impulsivity (e.g., difficulty organizing work and completing tasks, difficulty concentrating, being easily distracted, making sudden decisions without thought of the consequences).

C. The symptoms of inattention and impulsivity result in some impairment in social or occupational functioning.

D. Not due to Schizophrenia, Affective Disorder, Severe or Profound Mental Retardation, or Schizotypal or Borderline Personality Disorders.

That category was dropped from the DSM-III-R published in 1987. Rather, an insert appeared that read:

314.00 *Undifferentiated Attention-deficit Disorder* This is a category for disturbances in which the predominant feature is the persistence of developmentally inappropriate and marked inattention that is not a symptom of another disorder, such as Mental Retardation or Attention-deficit Hyperactive Disorder, or a disorganized and chaotic environment. Some of the disturbances that in DSM-III would have been categorized as Attention Deficit Disorder without Hyperactivity would be included in this category. Research is necessary to determine if this is a valid diagnostic category and, if so, how it should be defined.

The fourth addition of the *APA Diagnostic and Statistical Manual* was published in 1994. This time ADD in adults was listed in a

157

section entitled "Usually First Diagnosed in Infancy, Childhood or Adolescence." According to the manual, diagnosis can be made with either of two sets of symptoms. The first focuses on *inattention*.

According to the DSM-IV, for an adult to be diagnosed with ADD, he or she must have had problems in six of the following areas for at least six months:

A. Fails to give close attention to details.

B. Has difficulty sustaining attention.

C. Often doesn't seem to listen.

D. Experiences problems with follow-through or finishing work.

E. Has difficulty organizing tasks and activities.

F. Frequently avoids and dislikes sustained-action tasks.

G. Loses things needed for tasks.

H. Is easily distracted by extraneous stimuli.

I. Is forgetful in daily activities.

The second set of symptoms focuses on *hyperactivity/impulsivity* and also requires six symptoms persisting for six months:

A. Fidgets with hands or feet or squirms in seat.

B. Leaves seat when expected to remain seated.

C. Experiences feelings of restlessness.

D. Has trouble engaging in leisure activities quietly.

E. Is "on the go" often or "driven by a motor."

F. Talks excessively.

G. Blurts out answers before question is complete.

H. Has difficulty awaiting turn.

I. Interrupts or intrudes on others.

158

The behaviors must be present before age seven; be present in two or more settings, such as, school, work, or home; and the impairment must be visible in social, academic, or occupational settings.

Three subtypes are noted in the DSM-IV. Each has a diagnostic code that must be used when dealing with insurance companies and other official agencies. The manual states that most individuals have symptoms of both inattention and hyperactivity/impulsivity. Often, however, one or the other pattern is predominant. For a current adult diagnosis, one of the subtypes needs to be noted.

> 314.00 Attention Deficit/Hyperactivity Disorder, Predominantly Inattentive Type. This subtype should be used if six (or more) symptoms of inattention (but fewer than six symptoms of hyperactivity-impulsivity) have persisted for at least 6 months.

> 314.01 Attention Deficit/Hyperactivity Disorder, Combined Type. This subtype should be used if six (or more) symptoms of inattention and six (or more) symptoms of hyperactivity-impulsivity have persisted for at lease six months. Most children and adolescents with the disorder have the Combined Type. It is not known whether the same is true of adults with the disorder.

> 314.01 (Attention Deficit/Hyperactivity Disorder, Predominantly Hyperactive/Impulsive Type) This subtype should be used if six (or more) symptoms of hyperactivity-impulsivity (but fewer than six symptoms of inattention) have persisted for at lease six months. Inattention may often still be a significant clinical feature in such cases.

Future revisions of the *Diagnostic and Statistical Manual* are likely to further modify these criteria.

The Three Faces of ADD

▼

Over the last ten years, I have had the opportunity to talk with hundreds of people who had been diagnosed with ADD and have reviewed many more cases. From this experience I began to notice that people demonstrated one of three distinct clusters of symptoms. To be sure, some people were a mixture of the three, but frequently one form took precedence over the other two, sometimes to the exclusion of the other two.

Besides the obvious significance of these types for purposes of evaluation, I came to realize that intervention also had to be tailored to a person's particular form of ADD. The forms dictated the modifications I needed to recommend. I also noticed that I could often predict the types of medication that would be useful when I knew the form of ADD.

▶ **Form 1: Outwardly Expressive ADD: The Active Entertainer**

In this type of ADD, feelings and behaviors are expressed openly and actively. Impulsivity, impatience, and hyperactivity are readily apparent to everyone around. Hypersensitivity is dealt with by being over-reactive, "acting out" behavior, blaming others, and generally pushing the pain and discomfort away. Organizational challenges are usually met with an unwillingness to even attempt to get the job done or a frantic embrace of every organizational system that comes along in a desperate attempt to do something about the problem.

People with Outwardly Expressive ADD are often successful in sales, entertainment, entrepreneurship, and any field utilizing quickness, high energy, and risk taking. Difficulties arise because of:

hyperactivity	spreading energy too thinly	impulsivity
over-achievement	wide mood swings	disruptiveness
high risk taking	repetitious tasks	frustration
long-term projects	blaming others too much	temper
wanting one's own way	maintaining relationships	reactivity

People with this form are often outgoing and quite likable. Others see them as "getting away with murder." If you have this type of ADD, you need structure. Without firm guidelines for constructive ways to get your needs met, you are likely to get very out of control. It is quite important to provide early guidance to Form 1 people so their talents can be utilized to their satisfaction. Over-control and heavy-handedness with people with this form usually creates chaos and highly reactive responses. Requesting works much better than ordering.

▶ Form 2. Inwardly Directed ADD: The Restless Dreamer

In this type, feelings and behaviors are not expressed outwardly. Rather, if you have this form of ADD, you are more likely to "stuff" your feelings, keeping them to yourself and blaming yourself for anything and everything that goes wrong. Rather than "acting out" what you feel, you may think about how you would like to act it out but don't actually do it. To others you may not appear impulsive or impatient. However, you may feel both ways within yourself. Your hypersensitivity is likely to leave you feeling wounded emotionally, creating depression because you don't do anything about your feelings. You are tempted to just give in to your difficulties with organization and not try to overcome them.

People with Inwardly Directed ADD are frequently successful

doing technical and hands-on work, trouble shooting, and creative endeavors; working in professions that provide service to others, such as teaching, counseling, and social work; and in outdoor activities, such as landscaping and forestry. Difficulties arise because of:

under-activity	self-blame	poor task completion
under-achievement	burnout	wasting time
over-commitment	indecisiveness	inability to end bad relations
procrastination	depression	

The most frequently undiagnosed group, people with this type of ADD often suffer the most damage because of their ADD. Depression is likely to be severe. A consistent structure is very important to people with this form of ADD as are opportunities to be expressive in the manner that fits. For example, building things may provide an arena for expression that is gratifying. Otherwise, the inhibitions to expressiveness may further isolate these quieter people with ADD. Over-control and heavy-handedness with Inwardly Directed ADD people usually creates emotional damage that can be quite severe. Encouragement and building self-esteem are important.

► **Form 3. Highly Structured ADD: The Conscientious Controller**

If you have this form of ADD, your feelings are probably not actively displayed, though your behavior may be quite expressive and, in fact, controlling. Impulsivity and impatience are usually expressed as judgments. Hypersensitivity tends to take the form of blaming and judging others, the system, or the lawmakers who put restraints and rules in place. You *must* work within a structure, feeling out of control if the structure is changed. This leads to excessive controlling behavior in relation to others and your environment.

People with Highly Structured ADD usually succeed in the military, aircraft piloting, accounting, computer science, financial planning, or any field utilizing attention to detail and precision within a fixed structure. ADD people who go into professions requiring a lot of education, such as medicine and law, usually are high in this category. Difficulties arise because of:

excessive talking	obsessive worrying	perfectionism
unstructured settings	temper	over-control
problems recovering from interruption	over-focusing	rigidity
being judgmental	over-organization	demanding own way
inability to cooperate	difficulty with negotiation	

Rigid and controlling, people with this form of ADD often are perceived as hard to get along with. Your perfectionism and inflexibility also tend to make it difficult for you to work on a team, enjoy life, and relax. Though you may do well in a high-ly structured setting, outside of that structure you are likely to experience chaos and feelings of being out of control. It is very important to encourage people with Form 3 ADD to find or create reliable, consistent settings in which to function. Keeping firm but supportive limits in relation to this type of ADD is imperative if relationships are to remain healthy and growth-producing.

Remember, you may be primarily one type or a mixture of two or all three types. Each type of ADD requires different intervention for successful treatment. Be aware of how your ADD manifests itself and be sure you work with clinicians and teachers who can be flexible in assisting you so you can be successful in coping and growing as an adult with ADD.

Learning to Live with ADD: Five Stages

▼

While mingling with over three hundred participants at the first conference solely dedicated to serving adults who have ADD, the light bulb went off in my head. As it did, tears threatened to escape for all to see. I was viewing the happiness, healing, and growth of adults who previously had been lost or wanting, or whose lives were in disarray.

All around I recognized people with intense emotions; happiness, sadness, anger, excitement, euphoria, peacefulness were being expressed. These wonderful people were experiencing different levels of awareness and understanding about their ADD. I began to realize that what I was seeing were the stages through which people go as they integrate information about their ADD into their daily living. Five distinct stages emerged.

Stage One could be called the "Aha, I have it," stage. "Finally I have an explanation for why my life is the way it is. There really is *something* different about me. But I'm not crazy, retarded, lazy, inadequate, or no good." This is a time of awakening. It's recognition that "there are others like me." "I'm not the only one." Shock, excitement, and euphoria are likely to accompany this time as well as an insatiable search for information.

Stage Two can be called the grief stage. Once the realization sinks in that there was a reason for not being able to live up to

164

potential, the hurts, traumas, and losses suffered because of ADD begin to surface. As the mind begins to recall the hundreds of incidents that were related to ADD, the emotions begin to react. Confusion, anger, "what ifs," and depression all churn, creating emotional bedlam. This stage does end, but first it is important to feel the emotions and grieve the losses in order to heal the wounds.

Stage Three involves seeking support and understanding companionship during the grieving stage. This stage could be called the family stage. Over and over at the Adult ADD Conference, I heard people say, "I've found my family. There are others like me. I plan to come every year to my family reunion." Not only can information and guidance be gained at such groupings, but all important emotional support can be obtained. "Coming home" to a place of unconditional acceptance heals the wounds of the past and supports the growth of the future.

Stage Four is characterized by seeking, exploration, and experimentation. It might be called the growing up phase. It's a time for trying things. With ADD factored into a person's life, suddenly everything looks different. Exposure to previously tried experiences is necessary in order to discover from the new ADD perspective whether you like or dislike them, can or can't do them, want or don't want to pursue them now. It's an updating of data in one's bank of life experience.

Stage Five means coming of age. It is surely a time for the unfolding of a new identity. It's a time to redefine values, honor talents and gifts, and love who and what you are. "I know who I am now. I believe in myself. I can do whatever I've discovered I like. I am me." Reaching potential is wonderful, beautiful, and heady stuff. It is also possible and real.

The integration of current information into the life experiences of innumerable people is opening the door for the development of a valuable resource known to each of us: individual identity. As differences are recognized and honored, not only will individuals' lives be made more pleasant, but the world will truly become a better place in which to live. Let us provide support through the five stages of healing and growth of those with ADD in a context of understanding and acceptance. Then everyone wins.

Sample Adult ADD Assessment Interview

▼

A two-part interview has proven to be beneficial in the assessment of Attention Deficit Disorder in adults. The first session is an interview covering childhood and adult behavior. Complete school and family histories are taken; histories of personal life and job experiences as well as parental histories need to be extensive. In addition, an ADD checklist is completed by both the person suspected of having ADD and the interviewer.

It has been found to be very helpful to have a "significant other" (spouse, parent, friend, etc.) present for the assessment portion of the two interviews. Adults with ADD sometimes will not see their behavior as problematic or different, and having another person present can be very helpful.

It is good to get the ADD person to tell the complete story of what happened during any particular incident. They have so often been blamed for their lack of control that they assume they are at fault and do things for no good reason. When the details come out, especially in a supportive, non-judgmental setting, another picture of the incident may appear. I also always ask about the *intent* behind an ADD person's actions. That often has the effect of gaining their trust and produces a fuller picture.

PART I

► School History

Attempt to gather as much information about school experiences as the client remembers, as far back as the client remembers. What was school like for them? (Fun, hassle, enjoyable, depressing, something to try to get out of?) Did the person get in trouble more than the average kid? Was there a lot of daydreaming? (Check to see if this was a label put on the child or whether the person intentionally sought to fantasize.) What was the daydreaming about? Was following what the teacher was doing easy, hard, etc.? (Was recess the best time of the day?) Did he "lose interest" in courses which in turn led to problems with them? Was the person the one who was always talking with others, a class clown, "picking" at others, having trouble staying seated? How involved were the parents in their school? (Up at school a lot at the request of the school? Prodding at home to get homework done? Making sure the child finished things?) If the person attended college, what major was chosen and why? What attention/concentration problems remained in college?

When ADD is present, symptoms persist throughout school. Many have much difficulty when they become adolescents. Key times that difficulties are likely to show up are 4th and 7th grades and at the beginning of high school and college. Each of these grades tends to present the person with a new level of complexity both cognitively and environmentally.

► Family History

In talking about family, I usually ask the person to tell me about his or her family, what it was like growing up, what relationships were like between him and her siblings and parents, how the parents got along with each other, and how the child fit into the lineup. Was there divorce, separation, family problems, fighting or violence, physical, verbal or substance abuse, or

168

other addictions (eating disorders, sexual addition, workaholism, spending problems, etc.)? Was the person abused: verbally, psychologically, physically (including being spanked a lot), or sexually?

Get the parent's history, in school, work, and parenting. Does one or both parents have a temper, short fuse, or spank first/ask questions later behavior style? (Remember, many parents will turn out to have undiagnosed ADD too.)

▶ Personal Life

A brief personal history of the client focusing on the personal feelings, relationships, pleasurable activities and hobbies, goals and desires in life, and hopefulness for the future is necessary. Many times ADD adults will experience an overall feeling of depression and lack of personal fulfillment. Relationships may be volatile and/or the person may have trouble maintaining long-term ones. Intimacy can be difficult for persons with ADD.

People with ADD frequently need to relieve the stress that accumulates for them in daily living. TV, video games, music, racing (cars), and anything that has a vibration or hypnotic repetition, including jogging, are prime candidates for activities. Check for addictive behavior also, such as overspending, eating disorders, athletic addition, chocoholism, or any behavior engaged in with a vengeance.

Another good personal question has to do with the use of free time. What favorite hobbies or activities are preferred? This tells you what makes the person comfortable, even the well socialized one, when he doesn't have to feel responsible to do what he *should* do. Often persons with ADD will engage in hobbies that do not require great attention for extended periods of time or that fit their particular form of ADD. Golfers with ADD make use of the high degree of structure required by the game. Thrill-producing activities like race car driving rate high, as does street basketball or cruising, which allows the person to change direction at will. Music, dancing, and performing to a beat are often associated with ADD.

► Physical History and Status

Take a brief current and past health history. Inquire about childhood ailments and physical habits with special attention to sleep and eating habits. Ask about chronic conditions of a mild as well as a debilitating nature. Ask whether the person has had falls. Pay particular attention to times when his or her head was involved, regardless of whether loss of consciousness occurred. Inquire whether the ADD-like symptoms began to occur after an illness or injury. (Then it's not ADD.) Should there be a question about other organic problems including infection, head injuries, or seizure disorders, neuropsychological or nuclear medicine testing may be required to obtain a clear diagnosis.

Take a complete history of drug and alcohol use with the person as well as the parents and grandparents. Encourage the person to be forthright. Include questions about diet pills and the results the person experienced after the use of prescription or street drugs. (It's not uncommon for a person to get instantly "smarter" or more organized when taking diet pills.) "Speed" and cocaine also can produce positive results for people with ADD. The side effects, however, preclude their use, as does their illegality. There seems to be a need for people with ADD to anesthetize their feelings. Alcohol and marijuana, though ineffective in the long run, are often used in excess to self-medicate.

► Job and Career History

Take a complete job history. Inquire about the person's interest in the job, which aspects were easy and which were hard and what the person prefers. A large number of people with ADD go into sales, the entertainment business, and outdoor work such as landscaping. Inquire about reasons for leaving any jobs. Be supportive so that the person is not threatened by the questions. Find out whether the person left voluntarily, was fired, or work ran out. Ask about the specific circumstances surrounding separation from the job. (Temper and organizational problems are not unusual with people with ADD.) Look for job hopping and multiple job experiences. Ask about how the person got along with supervisors and what kinds of people the person liked to work for. Many people with ADD have problems with overbearing authority and critical types of management. They work best with positive, supportive reinforcement. Threats get nowhere and usually will cause an ADD person to bolt.

▶ Parent Interview

If parents are available, interview them with regard to the preschool years. Begin in infancy, especially with sleep, eating, and comforting patterns, response to noise, change, mobility habits, and physical conditions including colic, allergies, and irritability. Ask about parent involvement in school, calls to the school, teacher complaints, and involvement with homework. Check out accident proneness, breakage around the house, relationships with siblings, and disruptive interpersonal relations between the person and other family members and other kids. (People with ADD tend to have difficulty getting along with others because of impatience, temper problems, short attention spans, and a tendency to have difficulty waiting their turn.)

▶ Spouse or Friend Interview

Get the observations of a spouse or friend. Cover behavioral, interpersonal, emotional, and interest areas. Ask for vignettes. You might say, "What is it like to do yard work with this person?" or "What's it like to sleep with her?" or "Tell me the story of the last time you two went shopping, or did your income tax together."

171

► ADD Checklist 1

(Ask for specific examples)

	Yes	Some	No
Often fails to finish things started	——	——	——
Often does not seem to listen	——	——	——
Easily distracted	——	——	——
Has difficulty concentrating on sustained-attention tasks	——	——	——
Has difficulty sticking to an activity, especially one not desired	——	——	——
Often acts before thinking	——	——	——
Shifts excessively from one activity to another	——	——	——
Has difficulty organizing work or becomes disorganized if not following a schedule	——	——	——
Benefits from a structured environment	——	——	——
Frequently calls and talks out, interrupting conversations	——	——	——
Has difficulty waiting his turn in group situations	——	——	——
Impatient	——	——	——
Excessively on the move, often falling asleep when still	——	——	——

	Yes	Some	No
Has difficulty sitting still or fidgets excessively	___	___	___
Has difficulty staying seated	___	___	___
Moves about excessively during sleep	___	___	___
Always "on the go"	___	___	___
Engages in more than one activity at a time	___	___	___
Very sensitive to rejection, teasing, criticism, and frustration	___	___	___
Shifts moods suddenly and unexpectedly but based on events	___	___	___
Hot temper that disappears quickly (doesn't hold grudges)	___	___	___
Frequent negative thinking after excitement	___	___	___
Hard to give and take soothing and holding	___	___	___
Is soothed and/or aided in focusing by use of TV, radio, or fan	___	___	___
Tends to blame others	___	___	___
Stand-up comedy tendencies	___	___	___
Responds to asking better than being told	___	___	___

Yes responses to 40 percent of the above is indicative of ADD in adults when accompanied by a history of these behaviors in childhood.

▶ ADD Checklist 2

A checklist that I find very useful in diagnosing ADD was developed by Dr. Kathleen Nadeau ("ADHD in Adults—Diagnosis and Treatment," *HAAD Enough*, Nov/Dec 1990, p.7).

Some signs of Attention Deficit Disorder in adulthood include:

1. Chronic forgetfulness

2. Problems with time management (problems estimating realistically how long a given task will take and then allotting that time to the task)

3. Tendency to take on far too many tasks or projects

4. Generally disorganized lifestyle—frequently late, rushed, unprepared

5. Difficulty managing checkbook and finances

6. Frequent moves and/or job changes

7. Tendency to speak without considering the reaction which may be elicited by their comment

8. Tendency to interrupt others in conversation

9. Difficulty controlling temper

10. Difficulty managing paperwork on the job

11. Chronic pattern of underachievement (i.e., bright, but didn't excel in school; less advanced in career than others with the same years of experience)

12. Pattern of establishing relationships with caretakers—maybe a spouse, roommate, or secretary who serves as memory and organizer

13. Pattern of periodic depression which may begin in adolescence

14. Difficulty in maintaining long-term relationships (may have multiple marriages)

15. Greater than average tendency toward substance abuse

16. Tendency toward impulsivity—may make major decisions such as car purchases, home purchases, or job changes without careful, long-term planning

17. Tendency to be either over-active or under-active, with a previous history of overreactivity

18. Low tolerance for frustration—tendency to overreact to frustration

19. Tendency to give up on difficult, long-term projects

20. Pattern of interests which are taken up, then dropped, often after the investment of substantial sums of money in the pursuit of each interest

21. Difficulty concentrating when reading

22. Difficulty handling demanding learning situations which may be required for job advancement

23. Pattern of achieving less than siblings, academically or professionally

▶ Observation

The interviewer needs to make careful notes with regard to physical and attentional behavior during the interview. Watch for subtle as well as flagrant signs. Shifting of weight, finger drumming, and foot swinging are often present in excess. A need to get up and move around may be present. Accommodation of these behaviors does not interfere with the assessment and is the only kind thing to do for the person.

There is likely to be considerable sadness and even pain associated with some of the childhood and, at times, adult memories. Feelings of loss, shame, and inadequacy are quite common. Understanding and compassion are called for at these times. Sometimes, the person has bought into the system that accused and criticized him with how he "should" have been able to behave. It is common for an adult with ADD to put himself/herself down as a child, saying, "I just didn't listen" or "I just didn't try hard enough." This is a case of the victim joining the perpetrator. It is important to make it safe during the interview for the person to be able to be honest about actually having tried as hard as he or she could.

PART II

This session covers the results of the information gathered in Part I. It is preferable to allow at least three days between Parts I and II. Ask the person if he or she has had any other thoughts or feelings since the assessment. Clear up any questionable areas or concerns that you may have. Then, if you feel that the person has Attention Deficit Disorder, provide a training and education group, a study skills group if the person is in school, and a medication check if desired by the person. All referrals need to be prescreened to be sure the professional has experience with ADD. Unfortunately many professionals don't and will either discount the condition or give inappropriate support. Traditional psychotherapy is indicated for the secondary problems associated with ADD such as depression and trauma. Any work with interpersonal skill building, tutoring, or personal trauma reduction must take into account the special needs of the person with ADD. Traditional methods simply fall short.

A report and referral letter is indicated and it s recommended that these be shared with the person, who is seen as a partner in the evaluation and retraining process.

A three-month follow-up is indicated.

Sample Clinical Report Summary

▼

*A*fter you have determined by an assessment with a diagnostician that you are wired in an ADD way, he or she will put together a report similar to the sample given here. With your permission, that report will be submitted to your therapist, doctor, employer, school counselor, or anyone you wish to see it.

The report cannot ethically be shared without your permission. (A sample release of information form is included on page 186.) You determine to whom you want the report released and why: You might want your psychotherapist to know so your ADD can be taken into account. You may wish to consult your family doctor about a medication trial. Perhaps you want your boss to work with you to maximize your work environment in order to improve your concentration; or, you might want your school professors to allow you extra time or a quiet place to take an exam. Finally, in many states, ADD is considered a disability that falls under the auspices of the state Rehabilitation Commission which could qualify you for retraining to do work that fits you better.

ADD is also currently acknowledged under federal law through the Americans with Disabilities Act. You can request and expect to be given reasonable accommodation because of ADD.

A Typical Report of an Adult with ADD

▶ Presenting Concern

Joe Smith, age thirty-three, married and father of a three-month-old son, requested an assessment for adult ADD because of job related difficulties. He complained of problems concentrating on sales reports, due weekly, that took him three times longer to complete than his fellow workers. He reported getting distracted by office noise, clutter on his desk and an inability to remain seated for the sixty to ninety minutes required to complete them. He also reported concern over his temper that flares anytime he feels someone is taking advantage of him. He reacts to slight, unintentional occurrences such as traffic errors by others and his wife's expectations that he be able to follow through on household chores.

▶ School History

Joe was repeatedly chastised in school for having difficulty completing assignments and for not staying on task. His IQ was consistently reported to be above average. He never worked up to potential. He disliked school and found great difficulty staying in his seat.

▶ Family History

Joe spoke caringly about his parents but got along better with his father than his mother who he described as having a temper like his. His father was easygoing and much easier for him to relate to. He and his mother would get into "spats," walk off from each other and five minutes later have forgotten the whole thing. His mother did many things in excess: eating, buying things on sale, and taking on volunteer jobs that she could not maintain control of. Many a project necessitated pulling all night duty, the night before it was due in order to achieve completion. But she was a creative person who had a heart of gold and he loved her very much. He had one sister who got real good grades and was calm, cool, and collected just like his dad. He and his sister have come to appreciate each other but he has always felt inferior and used to wish he could be like her to get the approval she received. He feels lucky that his parents let him spend summers with his grandparents where he could be outside most of the time, running free and doing physical work.

► Personal Life

Joe loves being on the go, is amiable except when his temper gets the best of him. He always wanted to be a vet because he loves animals so much but never seemed able to pull the grades required. He knew he was bright enough but just couldn't settle down. He loves music and watches a lot of TV. These both help him settle down.

Joe's wife helps him a lot, loves him, and is described as very organized. He loves his baby and would rather spend time playing with him than doing chores.

► Physical History

Joe was a full-term baby who suffered colic from about two to six months of age. He has a history of allergies to many plants and trees, some foods, and cats and dogs. (He does own pets but they mostly stay outside.) There is no history of head trauma, serious infectious illnesses, or seizures. Generally his health has been and is good with his last physical two years ago. He did have a broken arm as a child from falling off a roof at age ten, as well as several severe ligament sprains from trying to climb trees and cliffs and from various and sundry other impulsive physical activities.

► Addiction History

When Joe was in high school he reports he drank too much but quit after a DWI scared him when he was twenty. He fears he could become addicted to alcohol easily. The only drug he experimented with was speed which he reported made him better able to focus on projects, but the side effects concerned him so he quit after a few months at age 18. Instead he drank. It didn't help his focusing but made him feel better temporarily from all the stress and fears of trying to get his life together.

▶ Job and Career History

When Joe couldn't make the grades to become a vet he tried several different jobs. He was happiest when he was around people and had the freedom to come and go as he pleased. He simply could not stand to sit behind a desk all day. He likes sales, but hates the paperwork. No matter how hard he tries, he can't stay focused on completing it. He intends to, tries to motivate himself, resolves every Friday to do better, and continually fails to achieve his goals. When it comes to making a sale, though, he's quite successful.

Mostly he has gotten along well with his bosses. The exceptions occurred when he was either yelled at and shamed in an attempt to get him to do something, rather than being asked, or when he had an excitable boss who continually changed his mind. (Though Joe likes variety and new things, he likes to be the one who does the changing. It confuses him when changes happen to him.) Joe reports functioning best when there is a regular, simple structure for him to work within that is not too demanding, has freedom but regularity.

▶ Behavioral History

Joe loves his car and wants to race. He says the thrill makes him feel great. He's trying to save his money now so that he can become more involved in racing as a hobby. He dreams of "being someone" someday. He wants his son to be proud of him.

Joe has learned to control his temper, tends to speed while driving, and must be "on the go" most of the time. He doesn't get into trouble for his behavior now.

▶ Spouse Interview

Joe's wife Anita reported that he tends to promise more than he can produce. She doesn't feel he intends to let her down, but he just gets distracted. Basically they have a loving marriage and both adore their baby, who was planned. She laughed that the hardest thing about being married to Joe was that he wanted to have the ceiling fan in their bedroom on winter and summer and admitted that he sleeps better when it is on than not. He is restless at night and at times flails out in his sleep. She's learned to duck pretty well. Fortunately they both have a sense of humor and good communication. She says Joe is never still for long, moving from one activity to another in the house. Sometimes they'll be in the middle of a conversation and he'll just get up and leave . . . not angrily, but he just goes into another room. If she follows him, he's very willing to continue the conversation, until he again moves to some other place. Usually he has gone to attend to some project or activity that he happened to think of while they were talking. At the movies, he drums his fingers and bounces his foot and often gets up at least once to get a drink or move around. In Sunday school, he is most comfortable sitting in the back of the room so he can get up during the discussion. She often notices him leaning against the doorway listening attentively. It's not that he isn't interested in the subject, he just can't sit still.

Joe's temper bothers her some, but she's learned that he gets over it quickly so she is less bothered than when they got married. Usually he reacts when he feels someone is blaming him for something or intruding in his space. She hopes he can get some help because she feels he is a real bright guy with a lot of potential if he can just pay attention.

▶ Observation

During the interview, Joe paid good attention the first ten minutes. Then he became restless, asked to get a drink of water after about twenty minutes and it was necessary to break the ninety-minute interview into several segments. Throughout the interview he jiggled his feet, drummed his fingers, and shifted his weight. He obviously is a well socialized, polite man who is cognizant of appropriate behavior and wants to cooperate.

Emotionally, Joe recalled many incidents in school when he was misunderstood and accused of not trying, when in reality he tried very hard. He said he always wanted to do better than he could do. He feels bad that he "caused his parents so much trouble." He never meant to. Now he's worried that he will fail his family because it's just so hard for him to get everything done that needs to be done. There is no indication that he doesn't want to do these things. He just keeps losing his attention.

► Summary

Joe Smith is a thirty-three-year-old married father of one who demonstrates numerous aspects of Attention Deficit Disorder. There is no indication that other physical or emotional abnormalities are present to account for his behavior. Joe can be expected to benefit from training to structure his life job and home projects. His wife will benefit from training to help her understand his needs and they can make tradeoffs to maximize each of their skills.

At work, record-keeping needs to be simplified for him. In addition, he may be able to track the records in a more beneficial manner during the week and his wife, in lieu of a secretary, may be able to help him complete the necessary paperwork in a more timely manner. He, in turn, is willing to take on one of her jobs for which he is more suited.

It has been recommended that Joe modify his diet with the help of a nutritionist. Particular attention needs to be paid to his tendency to consume candy and coffee, especially when he is frustrated doing paperwork.

Joe is being referred for a medication assessment.

He is also being referred to a training and education group for temper control and negotiation skill-building and to remediate the guilt and frustration he experienced growing up because of his ADD.

Follow-up is recommended at three months.

Model Letter to
a Physician

▼

To Whom It May Concern:

Patient's Name_____, has been evaluated for Attention Deficit Disorder at _____ Center. We have done an evaluation and found that he/she meets the criteria for adult ADD. (You may wish to list the form of ADD and diagnostic code here.) A copy of his/her report follows.

The research indicates that for some ADD adults, medication can be a significant benefit. We have informed him/her of this and have made a referral to your office for follow-up.

(If the physician is not familiar with ADD in adults you may wish to say . . .) Enclosed is some information to further familiarize you with this topic. We will continue to provide training, education, and counseling in relation to coping and accommodating the ADD.

We look forward to working with you and will provide you with follow-up periodically. Please let our office know of your treatment plan. Do not hesitate to let me know if we can be of further help to you at this time.

Yours sincerely,

Sample Permission To Obtain and Release Information

I hereby grant permission to _____
to request and obtain reports of psychological and psychiatric
evaluations and/or medical, school, social, and/or other appropriate records pertaining to:

_____   _____
(Name)   (Birth Date)

Permission is also granted for ___ _____ to
share findings, reports, and/or other information that might be
helpful in the understanding and treatment of this client with
other professionals and insurance companies if requested for
processing your claim.

The signer recognizes and agrees that a copy of this form is
acceptable and binding and will serve as an original in any
instance.

_____   _____
(Date)   (Name)

                             _____
                             (Relationship to Client)

Attention Deficit Disorder in Adults Workshop

▼

A three- to four-hour public workshop can be an invaluable community, college, or business tool to assist with initial identification of Attention Deficit Disorder in adults. There is a high level of accurate self-referral from this group of people.

At least two breaks are advisable, as well as an opportunity for people to move about, stretch, listen to a speaker for a while, then fill out the checklist and have small group discussions. Variability in format is essential.

I.   Introduction and Overview for the Day

II.   Content

    a. Screening checklist—to be filled out by each participant with regard to self or another

    b. What Attention Deficit Disorder is—attributes

    c. More complete assessment procedures

    d. Diagnostic criteria and complications, dual diagnosis

    e. Positive attributes

    f. Coping options

    g. Medication

    h. Resources in local area

      i. Success cases

      j. Living with ADD—special problems from the point of view of the significant other

III.   Questions and Answers

      Though questions and answers will be entertained throughout the workshop, they will be restricted to items of clarification since much of the material will be covered automatically. This section will be open for remaining questions and specific, personal questions.

IV.   Handouts will include:

      a. Checklist to be filled out

      b. A list of attributes

      c. A list of references

      d. A list of local and national resources

Running an ADD Group

▼

*I*n the education and training of adults with Attention Deficit Disorder, I have discovered a fairly short group series works the best. Similarly, it needs to run for a limited time period to hold the interest of the participants. This group is led by people who have a solid, practical, working knowledge of ADD in adults and good group facilitator skills. This group, based on a curriculum I've designed, is different from a support group in terms of intent and format.

Time: Four weeks (adolescent group, eight weeks preferred); two to three hours. I've discovered that shorter groups work well with the private sector, while longer groups are needed for those who have fewer life and living skills or who must deal with chemical dependency or incarceration issues.

Format: Get acquainted time followed by presentation of information and group discussion. Personal examples, question and answer time, and special needs included.

Leadership: The group can be led by a mental health clinician, educator, or group leader trained in the area of ADD in adults. I've developed a Training of Trainer's Curriculum specifically for people who want to run this group. See p.____ for more information.

Week 1:   Add fifteen to thirty minutes for registration, refreshments, and get acquainted time.

a. What it's like to be ADD. Presentation by peer leader is especially effective here.

b. Input by participants as they air their concerns about having discovered they have ADD. Personal stories are much in order here.

c. Participants list special problems they are facing on paper so leaders can be sure to incorporate solutions into future meetings.

d. A brief discussion of medication use often arises during this first meeting and referrals can be made for medication assessment.

Week 2:   Handling feelings

a. Present and past feelings need to be elicited from the participants.

b. Grief work is essential in helping people with ADD grieve for the losses incurred because of ADD.

c. Impulse and temper-control techniques are taught.

d. A stress reduction/relaxation technique needs to be taught.

Week 3:   Organizational management skills

a. Each participant needs to bring home and work examples of time management problems. Schedules are worked up and scheduling structures developed as date books and charts.

b. Ways to break up time are shared so that the person is more "in control."

c. Permission is given for each participant to do

whatever is necessary timewise in order to be successful. This includes leaving things to the last moment, working with the TV on, etc.

d. Spatial management changes are developed including the use of work carrels and other ways to break up space for more effective concentration.

e. Brainstorming is used to assist individuals to develop solutions to complicated situations. A letter may be developed for an ADD person to take to his or her boss or manager requesting special work arrangements. (A boost in productivity is quite appealing to many employers, particularly if it is only a matter of a fairly minor adjustment that makes the difference.)

Week 4: Interpersonal relations

a. Participants share specific problems they are confronted with in their relationships at home and at school.

b. Communications training is presented and practiced to help ADD people get their needs met and, in turn, to meet the needs of those with whom they interface.

c. Managing the "Uh-huh" phenomenon is taught.

d. Negotiation skills are outlined and practiced.

e. This final week ends with an appraisal of the question, "Who am I if I am in charge of my life and in control of my ADD?"

Medication and Attention Deficit Disorder in Adults

▼

▶ Interview with T. Dwaine McCallon, M.D.

When it comes to medication for adults with Attention Deficit Disorder, I have seen a wide range of awareness by physicians. Though pediatricians have prescribed medication for children with ADD for many years, few doctors are trained in or comfortable with prescribing it for adults. So, for more information on this important issue, I decided to talk with a professional whom I respect about medication and Attention Deficit Disorder in adults.

Dr. T. Dwaine McCallon, a Diplomate, American Board of Pediatrics, 1966, practiced pediatrics for eleven years before adding the treatment of adults to his professional experience. From 1977 to 1993 he maintained a private practice in rural Colorado in both general medicine and pediatrics in which he treated children and adults with ADD. During this time, from 1979 to 1993, he also gained experience as a part-time corrections physician.

Since June of 1993, Dr. McCallon has practiced medicine full-time in Colorado's largest prison facility. He is currently the Assistant Chief Medical Officer, Colorado Department of Corrections. During his tenure as a corrections physician, his treatment of Attention Deficit Disorder in adults has evolved and his understanding of the problem has increased significantly. I'm happy to be able to share his experience with you.

LYNN WEISS: What is most important to consider when talking about medicating adults?

T. DWAINE McCALLON: Accuracy of diagnosis is of utmost importance. A childhood history of ADD must be present. In addition, the DSM-IV criteria, published in 1994, must be met. A history of any reaction to medication treatment in childhood ADD is useful, as well as knowing about any adult or childhood responsiveness to mildly sedating drugs, such as anti-histamines. What we are looking for there is paradoxical response with over-activity or the reverse, over-sedation, with such stimulants as Sudafed or caffeine. Finally, an understanding that medicine is only one part of the treatment is crucial.

LW: What drugs do you consider using for the treatment of adults with ADD?

TDM: Ritalin (methylphenidate), Cylert (pemoline), and the classic Dexadrine (amphetamine) come to mind first for treating adults with ADD, as well as children. I also consider Catapress (clonidine), Pamelor (nortryptoline), Elavil (amyltriptoline) on occasion, and more recently Prozac (fluoxetine) and Wellbutrin (bupropion). The newer more specific or target-type tricyclic antidepressants have been found to be useful. And not to be forgotten is Tofranil or Imipramine.

Buspar (buspirone) is a non-benzodiazapine (non-Valium class) drug developed for the treatment of anxiety and has been found effective in a number of adult ADD patients. Although there have been reports that it may relieve levels of anger in certain patients, I have had the opposite effect reported by nearly half of the patients for whom I have prescribed Buspar. They have expressed fear that their feelings of control over their anger are actually decreased and that they might be unable to control angry impulses. Additionally, I have not been convinced that this drug is nearly as effective as many other medications for inattention.

LW: How does a physician know which medication to use?

193

TDM: Ritalin is still considered the "gold standard." The choice of agents can be effected by other presenting problems. For example, Pamelor is a very effective anti-depressant agent, as is Prozac. In the presence of a depressed patient with adult type ADD, one might take advantage of the effectiveness of Prozac on the depressed state and choose such a drug to treat both ADD and the depression. Another example would be the use of Clonidine in pre-treatment or treatment in the presence of broadened concept Tourette's Syndrome with attentional problems.

I have learned to warn my adult patients who display a lot of foot tapping, shrugging, finger drumming, and other so-called "excessive non-specific motor activities" about the possibility of Tourette's. Recently I warned an inmate in our prison to be sure and let me know if he felt an urge to swear when he didn't want to or anticipated "going off" (prison slang for losing control of temper). His reply was interesting: "How in the heck do you decide you're swearing too much in this place when every other word is _____ or _____ or _____!?"

Within two hours of his first dose of Ritalin, I received a plaintive note from the isolation unit, "Please tell Dr. McCallon to come get me bailed out of the hole. I think it's his fault I got here this time!"

When a corrections officer asked him how he was doing, this usually pleasant fellow answered with a diatribe of profanity that was amazing to everyone. He had also developed a one-sided mouth twitch, which was interpreted as a threatening posture.

Subsequently, we treated him first with clonidine, then cautiously added pemoline (Cylert) in a very small dose. At present he is working very well in saddlery and taking small business management courses successfully. He has stopped swearing and has had no violation write-ups in five months.

Another difficult therapeutic choice can come with treating

adult ADD in the presence of anxiety, anger, obsessive compulsive tendencies, or any combination of these.

To illustrate, I'm reminded of another recent case of an engineering draftsman who compensated for his ADD with rigidity and inflexible routines to accomplish his work. When his routine was interrupted, he became first anxious, then extremely angry. "I know they are going to foul up my project, and I simply told them off to get them away from my desk and my project" was his explanation. Closer questioning revealed a continuing anxiety and fear of "goofing up everything I try," which actually was a lifelong fear based on past failures.

Initially, I prescribed Buspar, which revealed the real stress—a fear of not producing quality work. This not only relieved the anxiety, but the secondary defensiveness melted, and the anger, to his amazement as well as mine, disappeared. Then we cautiously added Cylert, and, over a period of three or four weeks, we found a dramatic improvement in his focus and productivity, while he also became a lot nicer for his co-workers to be around.

He recently reminded me of something I told him at the beginning of treatment: "I think you are going to like you when you really get to know you without all of the symptoms of your ADD." His comment was, "You know, I really thought you were nuts, but you were right. I think I really like myself a bit now."

The presence of obsessive traits indicates that a therapist needs to look carefully for another congenital or inherited disorder, that is, pervasive Obsessive-Compulsive Disorder (OCD). Some of the newer mood-altering medications (including Prozac and, most notably, a drug called Anafranil) have been very successful in treating this condition. With what we are discovering about the brain chemistry in all of these states, it will be exciting to watch the development of more specific "target" drugs in the future. These are drugs very targeted to the area affected by the compounds within the brain and nervous system. The more specific and targeted a drug is, the less the side effect profile. One reason Ritalin is generally one of the best, if not *the* best, medication is because of its narrow effect or target. It has fewer side effects, which makes it a poor choice for treating depression.

Finally, in choosing a drug from the physician's point of view, the particular patient and his constellation of symptoms and whether or not he needs any medication at all has to be considered. Of course, side effects showing up in a particular patient may lead to a change in medication.

LW: What kind of physician should a person go to for treatment of ADD?

TDM: Any physician who is comfortable with ADD and familiar with the medications used to help it may prescribe the drugs. Family physicians in some instances are familiar with them, occasionally an internist is, and often a family pediatrician may be aware of ADD and comfortable in treating it. Moreover, neurologists are becoming more and more aware of and familiar with this disorder.

LW: Please discuss the trial and error approach to selecting a drug. How long does it take to get used to medications for ADD, and how long should it take for the drugs to take effect?

TDM: The choice of the use of medication and the particular medicine lies finally with the response of the individual to the drug used. Sometimes only a therapeutic trial will answer whether a particular patient will respond or not. On the other hand, a positive response really helps in proving that the diagnosis is ADD, if there had been any question regarding diagnosis.

Usually a response will be seen within two or three weeks, and very often it is seen in the first two or three hours with an amphetamine or methylphenidate (Ritalin).

LW: What problems confront physicians who prescribe medication for ADD?

TDM: Becoming familiar and comfortable with the condition itself, learning which questions to ask, and finding out if the medication is indeed helping the patient are necessary. Learning what side effects to watch for with each medication is also important.

LW: How often should a patient expect to be seen once the drug is stabilized?

TDM: Once every three to four months is usually necessary. Some of the medications are controlled substances and only one month's supply can be prescribed at a time. A tickler [computer reminder] file becomes necessary for the physician to write the monthly prescription and also is a nice way to be reminded to call and monitor the patient's progress.

LW: What are some signs that the drug is working?

TDM: Almost universally there is an ease and increased efficiency in dealing with tasks, as well as retention in reading. There's more understanding in reading something for the first time, especially if the patient is reading in a noisy environment.

Second, patients frequently report increased ease in understanding other people's conversations, especially in a noisy workplace or restaurant. Even on the first day patients often report that they can understand friends talking across a table or in a chair adjacent to them in a noisy environment. Very noticeably this is a pleasing sign that the medication is working.

Third, I hear fewer reports of problems with what is called *social, perceptive awareness,* in which the person jumps into action or talks before thinking. Less interruption of other people's conversations occurs. I've had two patients within the last three weeks report that they finally realized that they'd been interrupting their friends during conversations, have become sensitive to that, and have found that they are received far more warmly by friends in conversations now that they have "learned to wait their turn."

Another finding that indicates we are on the right track with medication in a patient can be seen with reports of greater levels of comfort working under pressure or in a demanding situation. Tasks are completed with less stress, too. There seems to be less flooding.

I've also had three patients in the last month who, since starting medication, delight in being able to use appropriate humor to make other people laugh. They like this newly found sense of humor.

Forgetfulness decreases, resulting in fewer mix-ups when shopping. This makes spouses happier. Prior to receiving medication, when asked to pick up something at the store, patients would either be distracted and forget to go or bring home the wrong item. After beginning medication, patients tell me, "I can remember two or three things I'm told to pick up, and I get it right."

Reduction in rates of "tool blindness" occur; that is, there is less loss of tools or pencils or books in the workplace. This is most impressive to the people with ADD who are mechanical and have good depth and spatial perceptions but who get very frustrated in having to repeatedly find the screwdriver or wrench.

A most delightful experience was pointed out to me by an engineer I recently started on medication. He reported an increased ability and sensitivity to sizing up other people's feelings in talking or working together with them. He realized why other people had disliked him. He had a great deal of difficulty in his workplace as a structural engineer. He had a history of being able to design bridges for the highway department but never received offers from the same contractor again because of his insensitivity to others. The most delightful part of this man's case was a report by his wife that he had become much more lovable and understanding now, a deficiency that he had been totally unaware of.

In our prison work a most dramatic change has been observed in about one half of our patients. This was first manifested as individuals telling their mental health counselor of a growing remorse and regret when they began contemplating the terrible effects of their criminal activity on their families and loved ones. One of our counselors has been bringing this out in group therapy sessions with adult ADD patients.

This introspection and developing awareness as well as concern about the long-term harm to others and themselves was the greatest surprise when we began screening and treating criminals. Taken with the increased social perception that we strive to create in sufferers of ADD, I feel this is one of the most exciting and important areas of self growth, one with tremendous importance for marriage, job, and personal success in all patients we are working to help.

The first patient in whom I saw this was a young man serving his third sentence. He responded to group therapy, counseling, and dramatically to Ritalin. Three weeks into treatment, he appeared for an appointment in serious remorse and regret but not in a helpless depression or thinking of suicide. This presented a great opportunity for building better attitudes and future behavior as he expressed his guilty feelings and deep regret at causing his mother and father such sadness as well as being an embarrassment to his sister, who is a college graduate and business owner. He is now laying plans to enter college and get his life in better order.

Fewer feelings of frustration occur when things don't go well. Finally, one thing that is quite diagnostic is an increase in legibility and neatness in handwriting. It occurs almost overnight with Ritalin, Dexadrine, or Pamelor.

LW: What if a patient thinks the medication isn't working?

TDM: Often people with ADD are quite pessimistic about medication. By being aware of what improvements can be expected with the use of medication, the physician can ask about these and help the patient evaluate the effects of the medication. Because of repeated failures in childhood, adolescence, and adult life, many people with ADD are so discouraged in their work and marriage relationships that they are actually frightened of again being disappointed when they think they may have found something that can help them get a handle on things.

Often a co-worker, supervisor, or spouse is very helpful in reporting dramatic improvements—that the patient is doubting—are actually occurring. By involving the spouse, we are often able to help the patient accept what is obvious to others. Usually, significant improvements show up in a number of areas.

In my experience, chronic failure and a mind set that expects a lack of success are the saddest and most tragic aspects of undiagnosed ADD, whether in adolescence or adulthood.

LW: What are signs that the drugs may not be working?

TDM: If there is lack of improvement in any of these areas, you can bet the drug is not working. One problem to be aware of is the inability to go to sleep readily at night, or worse, insomnia. This is often a symptom that the medication has worn off, rather than a side-effect of the medication. Another medication needs to be used that has longer acting properties which will last into the evening.

Other problems to be aware of include undiagnosed Tourette's Syndrome with involuntary, compulsive swearing, which can be a problem in the social setting. Some anorexia may be seen if the dose is incorrect. A few patients will report decreased control of anger. This has to be addressed very quickly. I warn the patient to let me know immediately if this happens.

Another problem occurs if the patient's mother used cocaine or crack cocaine when the patient was still a fetus. An Attention Deficit Disorder develops that is not responsive to almost any type of treatment. This is also sometimes seen with fetal alcohol syndrome.

LW: Talk about dual diagnosis.

TDM: One of the most difficult dual diagnoses I see involves what is called *broadened concept Tourette's Syndrome*, which is manifested by either involuntary animal-like sounds in adolescents and children or involuntary swearing. Sometimes, if this has been controlled by the patient, placing the person on a mild stimulant medication to treat his ADD will bring it out, along with facial or other body twitching or tics. If I find that a person seems to be rather hyperactive in adulthood, I very carefully warn them to watch out for these symptoms. Quite possibly, their medication will need to be changed.

Another common dual diagnosis involves tremendous feelings of inadequacy and worthlessness, previous childhood abuse, or a history of having been labeled a difficult child. I recently had a very tragic young man, nineteen years old, who sincerely described himself as a "meathead." When I asked how he had come to that conclusion, he said that was what his mother and father called him, and he decided that it was true because he could never do anything right. With mental health counseling, group therapy, and a low dose of Ritalin, this young man is now making a 3.6 grade point average carrying fourteen hours of college credit, while he works over thirty hours at an outside job. He is finally beginning to realize that he is not a "meathead."

This problem of low self-esteem and feelings of worthlessness are not only one of the most tragic parts of undiagnosed ADD, they also present one of the greatest difficulties in the diagnosis by providers not familiar with adult ADD. Many ADD patients are falsely labeled with bipolar disorder or manic-depressive disorder. The joyfulness and excitability that accompanies many types of ADD causes them to seem too euphoric at times while, because of the lack of success in their lives, they become depressed at other times. Because of the alternating periods of depression of happiness and hyperactivity, they are misdiagnosed.

Many of the inmates coming into our prison system are mislabeled in this way. They have every reason to be depressed, having "screwed up their lives" and ended up in a prison setting. This leads to a lot of depression. On the other hand, there are times when they are joyful, euphoric, excitable, and very talkative. They appear to the untrained eye to be overly euphoric and are, therefore, mislabeled as having bipolar disorder.

The most rare dual diagnosis that mimics Attention Deficit Disorder is minor-motor seizures, particularly petit mal or absence seizures. Careful observation of the patient during examination and evaluation should reveal this and careful questioning should readily separate this from ADD. If there is a question of a differential diagnosis, then these patients lend themselves readily to sleep-deprived brainwave studies with strobe light stimulation and hyperventilation to make a diagnosis.

LW: If a person has a history of drug or alcohol abuse, what are your thoughts regarding the use of medication?

TDM: The history of specific drug abuse is often very helpful in confirming the diagnosis of adult ADD. One constant in our prison population has been the pattern of drug abuse with unrecognized self-medication on the part of the patient. Almost all have chosen drugs with sedative or euphoric reactions, such as narcotics, marijuana, alcohol, even heroine. Almost all report they did not like amphetamines, as they did not obtain a drug rush or euphoria except at very high dosages. They did not particularly care for the calming effect of the stimulant at usual dosage levels.

In a great proportion of cases, patients reported decreases in their cravings for street drugs when on appropriately selected medication for ADD with conservative, small, frequent dosing. It appears that the stimulant drugs are helpful when given in small doses and selectively enhance the portion of the midpart of the brain that is involved in focusing attention, learning, and recall. In higher doses, the front part of the brain, the cerebrum, can indeed experience stimulation or "rush" in the higher centers, which is hazardous in addictive personalities.

Recent studies indicate that all the drugs that have been found to assist in ADD produce one or both of two hormone-like brain chemicals which are naturally produced in lower amounts in ADD patients than in people without attentional problems. The mild stimulant medications appear to cause the brain to produce more of these chemicals and so improve attention focus as well as speed of learning. This would seem to be the case in the majority of Attention Deficit Disorders. However, there is more than one type of ADD medication, and there are some types of ADD that are not responsive to medication.

In our early studies in a prison population with a very high level of street-drug abuse, the most encouraging finding has been that almost all of our patients have not asked for increased doses, but in many cases have actually asked to try lower doses because they have had such tragic results from illicit drug use in their lives. This has been so constant that an occasional request for more stimulant medication leads us to question the diagnosis of ADD and to re-evaluate the patient.

Frequently, the craving for drugs disappears in our prison population once appropriate medication for ADD begins. This is one of the most encouraging uses of medication in our setting.

LW: In addition to medication, what else do you feel people with ADD need in order to get their condition under control?

TDM: Medication is but one of many parts involved in understanding and getting ADD under control. Although in selected patients it is very useful, it is not the greatest part of the treatment. The five steps to directing and treating ADD covered in your book are most important, particularly the fifth step of maturation and growth in social and work skills as one discovers the delayed potential or, as you term it, discovering oneself. We see that with great gratification in our prison population as well as my private practice.

Family, employment, and learning areas demand treatment, understanding, and combined effort. Medication at best speeds the learning curve and is certainly not a cure-all for any type of ADD.

LW: Do people who are taking medication for ADD need to continue to take it their entire lives?

TDM: In some cases, lifelong medication for ADD may be needed. However, the goal should be controlling of one's life, of which ADD is only a part. With that control and mastery of the condition, medication-free success can often be obtained after two or three years. Intermittent medication for demanding situations may be indicated in a few cases, such as college exams or paper work involving an intense attention focus for a short period of time.

LW: Is it necessary to use medication if a person doesn't want to?

TDM: Absolutely not. Changing one's work and study habits as well as learning more efficient ways to accomplish goals, such as dividing work into small and manageable bits, can be very effective. Rehearsal of social skills before meeting new people or facing new situations may sharpen social perceptions. Faux pas and impulsive verbalizations that can be an embarrassing part of ADD can be avoided.

Many of the neat tricks described in your book can be built upon when the patient becomes aware of his disorder. The only limit is the persons' creativity. One of the pluses of ADD is the creativity that is a part of it.

LW: Can medication *cure* ADD?

TDM: No. It is only a part of the mastery of this very fascinating condition. The key is understanding and using the creative, artistic, or even humorous parts of it to build on so that ADD becomes one's attention deficit *advantage* for success and happiness. This is the happiest of outcomes in my view.

LW: What can people do if they cannot find a physician who knows about ADD in adults or is willing to provide medication?

TDM: The patient can start by learning everything possible about his or her ADD. If necessary, rehearse and then ask your physician to become more knowledgeable about ADD. If this fails, ask for assistance from mental health persons or clinics in your area. Find other people with this very common condition and begin a support group. Invite guest speakers and ask your own physician to attend and learn. Ply the doctor with literature. Travel to centers for consultation and then ask the consultant to send back reports with the reasons for the diagnosis and treatment recommendations, whether your physician has asked for it or not. Ask him or her if it's been necessary to change the thinking about ulcer disease in the last ten years, since we have found the bacteria that causes ulcers in most cases. Tell him ADD, a so-called behavioral disorder, is now known to be an inherited condition in most cases and is very treatable, and that he/she should learn more about it because treatment can be very successful.

LW: Do you know of any sources for obtaining ADD medications at a reduced cost if a person doesn't have the money?

TDM: This varies from state to state. With more class action suits to force school districts and boards of education to acknowledge and provide for this most common of the low-severity learning disabilities, I personally think that it will become acknowledged and provided for by medical assistance programs. County level social services may offer some funding.

LW: How do you feel about a person asking for medication because he or she thinks ADD is present?

TDM: I try to be objective with self-diagnosing. I determine whether the person has ADD and what type. I try to see how successfully the person accommodates it. I review job success and mental comfort, marriage stresses, and self-image. If the diagnosis of ADD is correct and I agree, I make very sure that the person understands what the medication is expected to do and more importantly what it cannot do. If I prescribe it, I have the patient back in two or three weeks to assess improvements that I expect and see whether we are getting them.

LW: What else would you like people to know about ADD?

TDM: Some of the most creative and delightful patients I have known are those with ADD. The tragic part is that they often do not believe or even know how intelligent they are, nor do they understand how delightful they can appear to others when they channel their good humor, artistry, and creativity once they have mastered their condition, turning it to their attention deficit advantage.

In my work in prison, I take great satisfaction in telling my patients, "I believe you are going to really like you when you get to know you." Then when they open the greatest Christmas present of all and realize they are not dumb or defective or lazy or "meatheads," the delight of watching this revelation unfold defies description. It is the most gratifying thing I have found in the practice of medicine.

Setting up an ADD Support Group

▼

A support group is a group of people who share a common problem and voluntarily come together for emotional support, information sharing (from those who are further down the road), resources, and problem solving.

You enter the group alone—you come out knowing you're not alone.

Support groups have the following characteristics:

Makeup: People who have a common problem but are at different stages of learning to handle it. Traditionally, support groups do not have a professional leader, though there may be an advisor. Specialists may be called in from time to time as speakers.

Desire: The individuals have a desire to solve or learn to live more effectively with their problem.

Scheduling: They tend to meet on a regular, predictable basis.

Politics: No one's vested interests are served by the group. It is not a way for one person to build business or in any way take advantage of the members. The group is organized for the purpose of assisting its members with the specific, identified problem.

To Start A Group:

▶ Check with your community's local service clearing-house to see if there is already one started, such as:

The Mental Health Association

An Information and Referral Service

or a national organization such as:

The National ADD in Adults Support Group (NADDA)

▶ Volunteer to serve as a contact person for others to call for information about a new group. Make a list of callers and get a couple of helpers. Find a place and set a date for the first meeting. Develop a network to get information out about the beginning group. Let the media and professionals know as they will make good referral sources.

▶ Meet with your local support group clearinghouse representative to get advise about starting and maintaining your support group.

▶ Consult a guide to support groups. An excellent resource is:

Helping You Helps Me: A Guide Book For Self-Help Groups, by Karen Hill. Canadian Council on Social Development, 1987.

Available from:

Canadian Council of Social Development, Publications, 55 Parkdale Avenue Ottawa, Ontario K1Y 4G1

You'll need to consider issues including:

▶ Generating membership

▶ Mutual partnership of support group and professionals

▶ Maintenance

    —balancing individual and group needs

    —leadership and control

    —agenda issues—support, education, activism, etc.

    —communication

    —confidentiality

Support groups can be wonderful. They can also get out of control and do damage to participants unless they are responsibly managed. If you become involved in a group that makes you feel worse rather than appreciably better, beware and look for another group or start your own. Don't hesitate to consult with a professional who is accustomed to dealing with self-help groups.

Organizations That Help Adults with ADD

▼

*T*he national ADD organizations vary with regard to what they provide people who are ADD and who work with ADD. Contact directly for more information. Many have national conferences that are excellent.

ADDult Support Network
c/o Mary Jane Johnson, President
2620 Ivy Place
Toledo, OH 43613

> The primary focus of this organization is to provide a national network for all adult ADD support groups, as well as information and support for adults with ADD. Mary Jane Johnson, president, was the inspiration behind the very first adult ADD conference in Ann Arbor Michigan, in 1993; was co-chair for the second adult conference in 1994; and was the conference chairperson for the National Attention Deficit Disorder Association's Adult ADD Conference in 1995 and 1996.

Support materials include:

- ► *Addult News* (quarterly newsletter): Personal stories, tips, news, open forum, conference/workshop information. ($15.00/yr.)

- ► *ADD-A Lifetime Challenge: Life Stories of Adults with ADD,* compiled and edited by Mary Jane Johnson. Each chapter is written by a different ADD adult. ($14.95)

▶ *Inside ADD-A Collection of Thoughts and Feelings on ADD,* by Susan Alfultis. The author's personal story, including journal entries, poems, and artwork. ($12.95)

▶ *ADDlibs and One-liners on The Lighter Side of ADD,* by Susan Alfultis. A booklet full of humorous ADD stories. ($6.50)

▶ The National Attention Deficit Disorder Association (NADDA)

NADDA was formed to unify and encourage ADD support organizations and to serve as a voice of national advocacy for ADD-affected individuals in matters related to health and education. The founders of NADDA came together in 1988 to work toward common goals:

▶ To represent and respond to the needs and concerns of existing ADD support groups. (NADDA is willing to exchange information and offer assistance. Materials have been formulated to assist groups in getting started.)

▶ To establish a public policy agenda to address statements and claims made about Attention Deficit Disorder through the media.

▶ For information on conferences write NADDA Adult Conference at address below.

Contact: National ADDA
           P.O. Box 972
           Mentor, OH 44061
           (800) 487-2282
           http://www.ADD.org

Materials: Write or call and request the ADDAlog, a catalog
            brochure listing NADDA materials for parents,
            teachers, adolescents, and ADD adults.

Addien (ADDult Information Exchange Network)
P.O. Box 1701
Ann Arbor, MI 48106

ADDIEN is a nonprofit support organization for adolescents and adults with ADD. Since 1993, ADDIEN has hosted the annual Adult ADD Conference. Each conference offers workshops and seminars on a wide range of ADD-related topics presented by nationally known speakers. A bookstore featuring one of the largest selections of books, audio and video tapes, and ADD-related material is also available. Regional conferences started in 1996, and the introduction of E-mail information is available from ADDinfo@ADDIEN.ORG. The Web page is at WWW.ADDIEN.ORG.

Contact: ADDIEN
P.O. Box 1701
Ann Arbor, MI 48106-1701
(313)426-1659 (voice mail)

CHADD
499 NW 70th Avenue, Suite 308
Plantation, FL 33317

A support group for parents whose children have ADD disorders, adults with ADD, and professionals who have an interest in Attention Deficit Disorders. The publications and activities often contain information about adults. CHADD sponsors a national conference and interrelates with national organizations forming coalitions that work for the benefit of children and adults with ADD.

Contact: (954)587-3700

Support materials available:

CHADDER is published two times per year in

journal/magazine format containing articles written by experts.

CHADDer Box, published monthly (except for summers), is a member's newsletter.

Learning Disabilities Association of America
c/o Jean Peterson, Executive Director
4156 Library Road
Pittsburgh, PA 15234
(412)341-1515
http://www.ldanatl.org

Adult Attention Deficit Foundation
132 North Woodward Avenue
Birmingham, MI 48009
(313)540-6335

Information/Resources

▼

*T*he following list is not meant to be inclusive nor should it be taken as a recommendation of professional skills.

► Newsletters and Handouts

ADDendum (for adult suffers of ADD)
c/o CPS
5041-A Back Lick Road
Annadale, VA 22003
(914)278-3022
Editor: Paul Jaffe, Legal Editor: Peter Latham, Esq.

ADDult News
2620 Ivy Place
Toledo, OH 43613

ADD Vantage
P.O. Box 29972
Thornton, CO 80229

ADDvisor
Attention Deficit Resource Center
P.O. Box 71223
Marietta, GA 30007-1223
Voice mail: (800)537-3784

Adult ADD Association
1225 E. Sunset Drive #640
Bellingham, WA 98226
(206)647-6681

Challenge Newsletter
c/o Jean Harrison
P.O. Box 2001
West Newbury, MA 01985
(508)462-0495

Med-ADD Services
P.O. Box 252
Boston, MA 02124
Editor: Peter D. Anderson, R.Ph.
(Pharmacotherapy and ADD)

The Attention Deficit Disorder in Adults Workbook

This companion volume to the best-selling *Attention Deficit Disorder in Adults* offers a combination journal, self-quiz, and organizer—all designed to give the user a daily, practical, hands-on method of living with A.D.D. Packed with more than 100 diagnostic self-quizzes, exercises, and daily schedules, *The Attention Deficit Disorder Workbook* is the essential guide for every adult with A.D.D.

This book retails for $17.95 and is available at bookstores nationwide.

A.D.D. on the Job
Making Your A.D.D. Work for You

Here is practical, sensitive advice for the employee, their boss, and co-workers and friends. Suggests advantages that the A.D.D. worker possesses, how to find the right job, and how to keep it. Employers and co-workers will learn what to expect from a fellow worker with A.D.D. and the most effective ways to work with them.

This book retails for $12.95 and is available at bookstores nationwide.